Behavioral Medicine in Primary Care

November 13, 2012

To Barry:
Here's to following
through with our
passions - career & otherwise!

Julie

Behavioral Medicine in Primary Care

A GLOBAL PERSPECTIVE

Edited by

JULIE M SCHIRMER MSW
Assistant Professor of Family Medicine
University of Vermont College of Medicine
Director, Behavioral Medicine
Assistant Director, Predoctoral Education
Maine Medical Center, Portland, ME, USA

and

ALAIN J MONTEGUT MD
Associate Professor of Family Medicine
Boston University School of Medicine
Director, Global Health Primary Care Initiative
Boston University, Boston, MA, USA

Forewords by
STEPHEN J SPANN MD

GABRIEL IVBIJARO MD

and

ALFRED LOH MD

Radcliffe Publishing
Oxford • New York

Radcliffe Publishing Ltd
18 Marcham Road
Abingdon
Oxon OX14 1AA
United Kingdom

www.radcliffe-oxford.com

Electronic catalogue and worldwide online ordering facility.

British Library Cataloguing in Publication Data

A catalogue record for this book is available from the British Library.

ISBN-13: 978 184619 357 6

Typeset by Pindar NZ, Auckland, New Zealand
Printed and bound by Cadmus Communications, USA

Contents

Foreword

The high prevalence of psychosocial problems in primary medical care practice is a global phenomenon. According to the World Health Organization (WHO), mental health disorders are among the leading causes of ill health and disability worldwide. Even the most developed countries lack enough specialized behavioral health professionals to deal with this burden of illness. No wonder the WHO has confirmed the need to integrate the assessment and treatment of mental health disorders into primary care.

While the principles and concepts of behavioral medicine are universal, their application in the care of patients must necessarily take into consideration the realities of the local healthcare system, and the patient's unique sociocultural context. Globalization has brought the need for cultural sensitivity and the opportunity for cross-cultural practice to many primary care practitioners around the world.

Health system reform in many countries continues to focus attention on the need for improving the quality of primary medical care. Specifically, an increasing number of countries are recognizing the need to train primary care physicians and other healthcare professionals deliberately through postgraduate residencies or on-the-job in-service continuing education programs in family medicine, for the purpose of developing a highly skilled primary care workforce. Specific, practical training in behavioral medicine is critical for these primary care practitioners.

This book fills a void by providing a practical, very readable "manual" for primary care practitioners to learn the fundamental principles and concepts of behavioral medicine and how to apply them to the local and patient sociocultural context. Edited and written by a group of healthcare professionals who have practiced and taught behavioral medicine and primary care around the globe, it covers a breadth of behavioral medicine topics with the depth needed by clinicians to provide competent care of the common psychosocial problems encountered in primary medical care practice.

The format of the book is very user-friendly. Each chapter begins with a brief introduction which establishes specific learning objectives. Each chapter has one or more clinical cases to illustrate the concepts discussed. There are multiple tables which are filled with practical information to be used in the clinical setting. Each chapter ends with a list of a few key resources which are available on the Web, as well as a useful list of references for further reading.

If you are a primary care practitioner working in a highly developed country with patients who have come from other countries and cultures, this book will help you better understand the cross-cultural nuances of behavioral medicine in caring for your patients. If you are a primary care clinician practicing in a country and culture different from your own, you too will find the book of great help as you practice in a cross-cultural setting. And if you are a teacher of primary care practitioners in-training anywhere, this should be an invaluable textbook for teaching behavioral medicine to your trainees. Wherever you practice or teach primary medical care around the globe, this book will help you provide better care to your patients.

Stephen J Spann MD, MBA
Senior Vice-President and Dean of Clinical Affairs
Baylor College of Medicine
Houston, Texas, USA
June 2009

Foreword

Behavioral Medicine in Primary Care: a global perspective provides the patient's story, enabling the patient's voice to be heard. It reminds us that people who consult primary care services are human and not just an illness and highlights the importance of social networks in well being and recovery by drawing on a decade of multidisciplinary expertise gained by working in primary care as practitioners and trainers in Vietnam and the United States of America.

The WHO World Health Report 2008 *Primary Health Care – Now More Than Ever* and the joint WHO Wonca publication *Integrating Mental Health into Primary Care: a global perspective* have already reaffirmed the utility value of the Alma Ata Declaration and reinforced the need for patient centred care. Patient centred care advocates that the best way to support the principles of holistic health-care is to enhance the application of the principles of the mind–body connection, stigma reduction, enhancement of patient strength and resilience, promotion of individual growth and recovery and harnessing of the patient's environmental and family support networks. Despite the recognition of these principles implementation of holistic patient care in practice has been limited. Patients seen in primary care settings are individuals who bring a complex mix of cultural, social, psychological, and biological factors that manifest in the consultation. Understanding and formulating these factors can lead to a true partnership between patients and care givers and allows for the ideas, concerns, expectations and cultural perspective of the patient to be aligned with those of the care provider to promote concordance and better health outcomes. This approach is core to the schemas adopted by behavioral medicine.

The authors of this book advocate practical ways of improving the recognition and implementation of patient centred care. They use a series of case vignettes as a lens for directing readers to a conceptual understanding of the mind and body and the relationship to the principles of behavioral medicine. They further crystallise the definition of behavioral medicine and describe three systemic models: the medical model, the public health aspect, and the traditional medicine model which enable the primary care practitioner to better understand the role of the cultural perspective in the formulation of problems presenting to primary care.

This book provides a range of questionnaires and checklists to aid primary care practitioners to implement principles and concepts from behavioral medicine to primary care. Application of the principles advocated by *Behavioral Medicine in Primary Care: a global perspective* will make a difference to patient outcomes, whatever country or continent that they live in.

Dr Gabriel Ivbijaro MBBS, FRCGP, FWACPsych, MMedSci, DFFP, MA
Chair of the Wonca Working Party on Mental Health
June 2009

Foreword

Over the past several decades, the practice of medicine has been increasingly fascinated with and influenced by high-tech developments and disease-focused approaches. This is especially evident in developed countries and even in some developing countries.

It is often forgotten that a significant percentage of patients seen in the family practice setting will not benefit from these latest advances. In cases where psychosocial and psychosomatic causations and manifestations of illness are the underlying reasons for the encounter with the family doctor, the application of behavioral medicine best practices may make all the difference in the outcome for the patient.

This book, on *Behavioral Medicine in Primary Care: a global perspective*, written by family physicians for family physicians, will in my view prove an invaluable resource for those who dare to take on the challenge of initiating behavioral change in their patients using principles and strategies proven effective in multiple countries and cultures. The approach the two co-editors have taken of having case scenarios at the start of each chapter to illustrate underlying strategies or principles is unique and refreshing. These case scenarios illustrate how behavioral medicine strategies can be applied in different healthcare systems and in the context of different cultural settings. Having contributions by primary and contributing chapter authors who are from or have had experiences in providing healthcare in different countries at varying levels of primary care development makes the book relevant in primary care settings in countries at various stages of development.

Mental health and behavior-related disorders are becoming an increasingly important aspect of total healthcare, as more developing countries emerge from the initial phases of their healthcare evolution, from the control of infectious diseases to chronic disease care and diseases of life-styles, and as more of the world's population migrate into urban centres. This book, when read in conjunction with the newly published *Report on Integrating Mental Health into Primary Care* by the World Health Organization (WHO) and The World Organization of Family Doctors (Wonca), together provide family physicians with an invaluable resource on behavioral medicine in primary care.

Dr Alfred Loh
CEO
The World Organization of Family Doctors (Wonca)
June 2009

Preface

This textbook provides primary healthcare practitioners with strategies for applying the principles and concepts of behavioral medicine to patient care. The idea for this book emerged from numerous conversations between the various authors in their decade-long experience of incorporating behavioral medicine principles into Vietnam's family medicine training programs. This team of US and Vietnam colleagues wanted a textbook that described how behavioral medicine principles could be applied to patients and healthcare systems in cultures different from the Western model of care.

Most behavioral medicine textbooks are geared towards Western cultures, which value autonomy and independent decision making about patient health, and where psychiatrists and other mental health professionals are available to care for patients and train healthcare practitioners. We wanted a book that would prepare primary care clinicians to care for patients when mental health and behavioral health specialists were unavailable, whether that care was provided at home or abroad.

We live in an increasingly multi-cultural world. In 2006, immigrants represented 12% of the population in the USA,[1] 18% of that in Canada and 9% of that in the UK.[2] As air travel has become more affordable and advances in telecommunication have made intercontinental relationships more feasible, physicians and other healthcare practitioners have been seeking training and practice opportunities in other parts of the world.

Our goal was to create a book that was comprehensive and practical, but not so detailed as to overwhelm all but behavioral medicine specialists. We wanted a textbook that primary healthcare clinicians would find inviting and interesting, and which would provide them with skills that they could immediately apply to patient care. Our definition of the term "clinician" includes anyone seeing patients for primary healthcare purposes, including physicians, assistant physicians, nurses, midwives, social workers, and healthcare workers in community health sites, private clinics, or in patients' homes.

The impact of behavioral health on biological health is well recognized. Unhealthy beliefs, behaviors, and lifestyle choices of people contribute to more than 50% of the conditions that are treated in primary care sites.[3] Clinical interventions by physicians and other healthcare workers have been shown to be effective in changing unhealthy behaviors in multiple primary healthcare settings with populations as diverse as vulnerable mothers in Pakistan, commercial sex workers in Asia, and smokers in Zimbabwe.

We recognize that a large proportion of health behaviors are determined by factors over which patients have little or no control, such as poverty, early childhood exposure to trauma, war, birth defects, and environmental issues such as lack of access to clean water. Although the majority of this book focuses on what occurs during the clinical visit, Chapter 6 discusses how practitioners can seek to address many of these issues by working with community groups.

In 2001, the World Health Organization (WHO) published a report which confirmed the need to integrate the assessment and treatment of mental health disorders into primary care. According to this report, mental health disorders are among the leading causes of ill health and disability worldwide.[4] Successful treatment of mental health disorders and assistance with stress responses and health-defeating behaviors help patients to adhere to treatment, increase their capacity to deal with pain and disability, and reduce their emotional and physical pain.

Nearly two-thirds of individuals with known mental health disorders do not seek help from mental health professionals.[5] Therefore all members of the primary healthcare team need the training and skills to assess and support patients with common mental health issues. Members of the healthcare team play different roles in assessing, counseling, treating, and referring patients for additional support. We have attempted to delineate these roles throughout this book wherever possible.

CONSTRAINTS

There are numerous barriers to the incorporation of behavioral medicine principles into primary healthcare practice. In countries with developing economies, behavioral health issues have a lower priority than basic needs such as food, clothing, and shelter. Resource-poor countries are constrained to apply healthcare resources to address infectious disease, malnutrition and only the most debilitating mental health conditions. As governments gain stability and their economies grow stronger, they can more easily meet the basic needs of the population and devote more resources to behavioral health issues.

According to the World Bank, Vietnam is classified as a low income country, where 25% or more of the population earn less than $1 per day.[6] This is the case in many countries in South-East Asia, and in almost half of the countries in Africa, where 25–80% of people live in such extreme poverty. Extreme poverty means that families have difficulty meeting basic needs such as food, shelter and healthcare.[7]

In countries with extreme poverty, there are shortages of trained medical practitioners at all levels. Many of these countries have no clear national strategy for dealing with mental health issues, other than institutionalizing the most severe cases. The roles of mental health and primary care practitioners may not be clearly defined, resulting in turf battles over who cares for patients with mental health disorders.

In many developing countries, primary care practitioners are not approved to prescribe psychotropic medications, and the medications are not available at the primary care sites. Ideally, in countries with limited resources, mental health specialists would focus more on consultation and training primary care practitioners, and less on seeing patients. For example, Belize has developed a national strategy, providing mental health training for nurses, who travel to primary healthcare sites around the country to consult on patients seen by the primary care practitioners and to provide training.[8]

ORGANIZATION OF THE BOOK

After the introductory chapter, all subsequent chapters begin with case scenarios that illustrate how the behavioral medicine strategies can be applied in different healthcare systems. Many of the cases show how the models, such as cognitive therapy, can be modified, depending on the system and culture. At the end of each chapter, two or three (sometimes more) key resources are listed, many of which are Internet-based, for those who are interested in learning more about the concepts described in that chapter.

Chapter 1 describes in detail the theoretical underpinnings and evidence that support the incorporation of behavioral medicine into primary care. It provides key definitions, core principles, and an overview of how the principles are applied in clinical care.

Chapter 2 begins with a case scenario that illustrates a very unsatisfactory doctor–patient encounter, with a patient whose physical complaint is limiting her functioning at work and at home. The chapter provides a history of the doctor–patient relationship in Western medicine, describes the difference between disease (the pathological process) and illness (the patient's experience of the effect of the illness on their health), and recommends core communication skills that primary care practitioners can apply when seeing patients.

Chapter 3 begins with two case scenarios about women who are each experiencing a different stress-related syndrome that is specific to Latin American and Asian cultures. The chapter uses these cases to illustrate the influence of culture and stress on the body. It delineates how the mind can help or hinder a person's reaction to stress, and counseling techniques that practitioners can use to help patients to change unhealthy ways of thinking.

Chapter 4 incorporates several case scenarios about patients whose behaviors are interfering with their health. Several behavioral change models and strategies are described and applied to help these patients with smoking cessation, problem drinking, and unsafe sexual practices.

Chapter 5 begins with a case scenario about a woman whose headache and fatigue symptoms are influenced by her family's adaptation to her husband's retirement and her mother-in-law's increasing physical dependence. It illustrates her family's influence on her health, and demonstrates multiple strategies that healthcare practitioners can use to assess and interact with families to improve their overall health.

Chapter 6 begins with two case scenarios about Somali mothers who are experiencing postpartum depression. The cases contrast the differences in perspectives and resources for patients living in rural and urban settings in the same country. The chapter describes the different categories of healers, and the different explanations of symptoms as seen by patients and practitioners. This material complements Chapter 3 in suggesting strategies for dealing with the different perspectives of patients and practitioners. It also describes community strategies that primary care practitioners can use to address the health issues of their patient population. Finally, this chapter provides strategies to enable practitioners to become culturally sensitive with their patients and to help to prepare them for working in countries other than their home country.

Chapter 7 begins with case scenarios about two patients, who are experiencing depression and substance abuse disorders. It suggests strategies for practitioners to use to assess and treat common mental health conditions, including depression, anxiety, somatoform disorders, sleep disorders, chronic fatigue, and substance abuse disorders. Screening questions and easy-to-use assessment tools are provided for many of the conditions.

Chapter 8 begins with a case scenario about a recently widowed mother suffering from extreme fatigue, who discovers that she is HIV positive. This case demonstrates the practitioner using a patient-centered approach to help the patient to adjust to this new diagnosis and deal with discussing the process and implications of having her daughters tested for the virus. The chapter discusses the elements of effective counseling, and counseling models that are practical for primary care practitioners.

Chapter 9 focuses on practitioner well-being, beginning with three stories of practitioners living in Central America, the USA, and rural Kenya. The chapter makes the case for practitioner well-being and self-care as important components of healthcare, delineating the pitfalls, the obstacles, and the steps to take in order to achieve optimal health of the practitioner and their colleagues.

Chapter 10 illustrates the strategies and principles that can be used to develop behavioral medicine in healthcare systems where the concepts may not exist and where there may be few trained behavioral medicine specialists. It demonstrates principles and strategies both through our work in Vietnam and through the many other successful international projects that are integrating mental health into primary care practices around the world.

Julie M Schirmer
Alain J Montegut
June 2009

REFERENCES

1 Grieco E. *Immigrant Union Members: numbers and trends.* Immigration Facts (Internet-based serial), 2004; www.migrationpolicy.org/pubs/7_Immigrant_Union_Membership.pdf (accessed 17 January 2009).
2 United Nations, Department of Economic and Social Affairs, Population Division. *International Migration 2006*; www.un.org/esa/population/publications/2006Migration_Chart/2006IttMig_chart.htm (accessed 18 January 2009).
3 World Health Organization. *The World Health Report 2002. Reducing risks, promoting healthy life*; www.who.int/whr/2002/en/ (accessed 18 January 2009).
4 World Health Organization. *The World Health Report 2001. Mental health: new understanding, new hope*; www.who.int/whr2001/2001/main/en/chapter2/index.htm (accessed 2 July 2004).

5 World Health Organization. *The World Health Report 2001. Mental health: new understanding, new hope*; www.who.int/whr2001/2001/main/en/chapter2/index.htm (accessed 2 July 2004).
6 World Bank. *Poverty Calculator Net*; http://iresearch.worldbank.org/PovcalNet/jsp/index.jsp (accessed 23 April 2007).
7 Sachs J. *The End of Poverty: economic possibilities of our time*. New York: Penguin Press; 2005.
8 World Health Organization. *WHO/Wonca Joint Report: integrating mental health into primary care – a global perspective*; www.who.int/mental_health/policy/Mental%20 health%20+%20primary%20care-%20final%20low-res%20140908.pdf (accessed 13 April 2009).

List of editors

Julie M Schirmer, MSW
Assistant Professor of Family Medicine, University of Vermont College of Medicine, Department of Family Practice, Burlington, VT
Director of Behavioral Medicine and Assistant Director of Predoctoral Education, Family Medicine Department, Maine Medical Center, Portland, ME, USA

Alain J Montegut, MD
Associate Professor of Family Medicine, Boston University School of Medicine, and Director of the Global Health Primary Care Initiative, Department of Family Medicine, Boston University, Boston, MA, USA

List of contributors

PRIMARY CHAPTER AUTHORS

Alan Lorenz, MD
Associate Professor of Family Medicine and Psychiatry, University of Rochester
  School of Medicine and Dentistry, Rochester, NY, USA

Daniel L Meyer, PhD
Public Health/Evaluation Consultant, Readfield, ME, USA

Alain J Montegut, MD
Associate Professor of Family Medicine, Boston University School of Medicine,
  and Director of the Global Health Primary Care Initiative, Department of Family
  Medicine, Boston University, Boston, MA, USA

Cathleen Morrow, MD
Associate Professor of Community and Family Medicine, Dartmouth Medical
  School, and Director of Pre-Doctoral Education, Dartmouth Medical School,
  Hanover, NH, USA

Julie M Schirmer, MSW
Associate Professor of Family Medicine, University of Vermont College of Medicine,
  Department of Family Practice, Burlington, VT, and Director of Behavioral
  Medicine and Assistant Director of Predoctoral Education, Family Medicine
  Department, Maine Medical Center, Portland, ME, USA

Jeffrey Stovall, MD
Associate Professor of Psychiatry and Residency Training Director, Department of
  Psychiatry, Vanderbilt University, Nashville, TN, USA

William Ventres, MD
Multnomah County Health Department, Mid-County Health Center, Portland,
  OR, USA

CONTRIBUTING CHAPTER AUTHORS

Kamlesh Bhargava, MD, MRCGP (Int)
Department of Family Medicine and Public Health, College of Medicine and Health
  Sciences, Sultan Qaboos University, Muscat, Sultanate of Oman

Nguyen Thi Kim Chuc, PhD
Associate Director of the Family Medicine Department at Hanoi Medical University,
  Hanoi, Vietnam

Pham Huy Dung, MD, PhD
Professor of Social Work at Thang Long University and Professor of Family
  Medicine at Hanoi Medical School, Hanoi, Vietnam

Ellen Fiore
Editorial Consultant, Harrison, NY, USA

Kimberly Green, MA
Senior Technical Officer, Asia Pacific Regional Office, Care and Support Division
  of Family Health International, Hanoi, Vietnam

Christina Holt, MD
Assistant Professor of Family Medicine, University of Vermont School of Medicine,
  Burlington, VT, and Director of Research, Family Medicine Department, Maine
  Medical Center, Portland, ME, USA

Nguyen Van Hung, MD, PhD
Head of Family Medicine Unit, Chairman, Department of Pharmacology, Hai
  Phong Medical University, Vietnam

Nguyen Vu Quoc Huy, MD, PhD
Director of International Affairs, Hué Medical College, Hué, Vietnam

Thich Linh, MD
Psychiatrist, Family Medicine Center, University of Medicine and Pharmacy, Ho
  Chi Minh City, Vietnam

Le Hoang Ninh, MD, PhD
Director of the Institute of Hygiene and Public Health, Ho Chi Minh City,
  Vietnam

Nguyen Duy Phong, MD, PhD
Lecturer, Department of Infectious Disease and Family Medicine Center, University
  of Medicine and Pharmacy, Ho Chi Minh City, Vietnam

Nguyen Van Son, MD, PhD
Vice Rector, Thai Nguyen Medical University, Thai Nguyen, Vietnam

Nguyen Minh Tam, MD, PhD
Lecturer in Public Health, Hué Medical College, Hué, Vietnam

Au Bich Thuy, MD, MSc
Lecturer and Secretary of Family Medicine, Can Tho University of Medicine and Pharmacy, Can Tho, Vietnam, and Researcher, Menzies Research Institute, University of Tasmania, Hobart, Australia

Le Than Toan, MD
Lecturer, Family Medicine Center, University of Medicine and Pharmacy, Ho Chi Minh City, Vietnam

Acknowledgments

Many people have contributed to the development of this book, which was written or reviewed by over 40 authors with experience in behavioral medicine as applied to primary healthcare in the USA and other international settings. We knew that this book could not be written alone, and also that it should not focus strictly on Vietnam. Our clinical and teaching experience in our home countries and from our work in Vietnam and other international settings could be instructional to others who are caring for patients, particular those from different cultural communities. We wanted to create a practical textbook that could provide readers with fundamental skills in behavioral medicine which they could immediately begin to apply to patient care. We incorporated case scenarios to allow readers to virtually "see" behavioral medicine in action in multiple countries and settings.

The primary authors of each chapter are all senior faculty in family medicine, psychiatry, or behavioral medicine who have taught or consulted in Vietnam. Many have consulting healthcare experience in other countries as well. The Vietnamese co-authors have added their stories and perspectives to each chapter, helping the US authors to better understand their issues and struggles. The writing of the US authors has in turn helped to increase the Vietnamese authors' understanding of the principles of behavioral medicine. This book could not have been written without the hard work and dedication of these Vietnamese physicians, who questioned, challenged, and integrated the behavioral medicine principles that worked best for them in their teaching and patient care.

To help to make the book as relevant as possible to multiple settings and learners, we sought ongoing reviews from students, residents in training, and experts in family medicine and behavioral medicine. We enlisted reviewers and co-authors who either were living in or had consulting experience in other international settings, such as Oman, Kenya, Lebanon, Niger, and Chile. We scanned the literature, looking for evidence that would indicate the relevance of the practice models in a range of countries.

The chapters were rewritten as necessary to incorporate most of the reviewers' suggestions. Val Hart, who has taught English as a Foreign Language for over 20 years, finally edited the text to make it more easily understood by readers whose primary language is not English.

So much has gone into the writing of this book that would remain hidden unless it was specifically recognized in acknowledgments such as this. Ellen Fiore was the person who really convinced us that this book needed to be written, and provided the initial instruction and vision on "how to eat an elephant, one bite at a time." Larry Bauer, Executive Director of the Family Medicine Education Consortium, strongly believed in the mission and the people involved in this project. He provided guidance and support when the momentum seemed to diminish, and he bore witness to and celebrated the successes of the book and the overall development project throughout the years. Laneay Yates dedicated her house and home to bringing together the myriad last-minute details in order to get the book published on time. Gillian Nineham at Radcliffe Publishing believed in our vision and guided us through the publishing process.

And saving our loved ones for last, William Schirmer, MD and Kathleen Montegut, MS APRN lovingly supported the actual writing of this book, caring for house and home during our consultation visits to Vietnam and other countries, providing late-night meals, and editing last-minute versions of text at weekends and during vacations. We understand and appreciate the sacrifices that families make to enable writers to fulfill their dreams.

We thank all of the many chapter authors, reviewers, and other individuals who provided support in a variety of ways, who together made the writing of this book possible.

REVIEWERS

Ray Downing, MD
Faculty of Family Medicine
Moi University School of Medicine
Eldoret, Kenya

Craig Van Dyke, MD
Professor of Psychiatry
Director of the Global Mental Health Program
University of California
San Francisco, CA, USA
Program Director (IPA)
National Institute of Mental Health
Rockville, MD, USA

Tim Gagne, MD, MPH
Medical Resident
Family Medicine Department
Maine Medical Center
Portland, ME, USA

Jason Goldie, MD
Medical Resident
Family Medicine Department
Maine Medical Center
Portland, ME, USA

Jeffrey Grassman, MD
Medical Resident
Family Medicine Department
Maine Medical Center
Portland, ME, USA

Brandon Green
Development Exchange Officer
American Medical Student Association
International Federation of Medical Students' Associations
Washington, DC, USA

Donna Kim, MD
Medical Resident
Family Medicine Department
Maine Medical Center
Portland, ME, USA

Richard G Roberts, MD, JD
President Elect, Wonca
Professor of Family Medicine
University of Wisconsin
Madison, WI, USA

Ed Shahady, MD
Medical Director
Diabetes Master Clinician Program
Florida Academy Family Physicians
Foundation
Fernandina Beach, FL, USA

Smita Sonti, MD, MPH
Medical Resident
Family Medicine Department
Maine Medical Center
Portland, ME, USA

Kenneth S Thompson, MD
Associate Professor of Psychiatry and Public Health
University of Pittsburgh and
Western Psychiatric Institute and Clinic
Pittsburgh, PA
Associate Director of Medical Affairs
Center for Mental Health Services
Substance Abuse and Mental Health Services Administration
Washington, DC, USA

CHAPTER REVIEWERS

William A Alto, MD, MPH
Professor of Family and Community Medicine
Dartmouth Medical School
Hanover, NH, USA

Richard J Botelho, MD
Professor of Family Medicine and Nursing
Director of Fellowship Training
Department of Family Medicine
University of Rochester School of Medicine and Dentistry
Rochester, NY, USA

Lucy Candib, MD
Professor of Family Medicine and Community Health
University of Massachusetts Medical School
Family Health Center of Worcester
Worcester, MA, USA

Paige Clark, MD
National Vice President for Membership
American Medical Students Association
Washington, DC, USA

Lilianna Rivis, MD
Family Medicine Physician
Waterville, ME, USA

Ovidio Rivis, MD
Psychiatrist
Waterville, ME, USA

Debra Rothenberg, MD, PhD
Assistant Program Director
Family Medicine Center
Maine Medical Center
Portland, ME, USA

Alex Tsai, MD
Medical Resident
Department of Psychiatry
University of California
San Francisco, CA, USA

EDITOR
Valentine Hart, MEd
Writer and editor (English as a Foreign Language specialty)
Language and Multicultural Resources
Cumberland, ME, USA

CHAPTER 1

Behavioral medicine: principles and practices

Julie M Schirmer and Le Hoang Ninh

INTRODUCTION

This introductory chapter provides an overview of the key components of behavioral medicine. This chapter provides the rationale and evidence that support the integration of behavioral medicine into primary care. The subsequent chapters are extremely practical, describing how the principles and concepts of behavioral medicine can be applied in healthcare settings in the USA and in developing countries. Although the focus is on family medicine and primary care, the principles and skills can be applied in community settings such as HIV/AIDS centers, palliative care clinics, and alcohol or drug treatment centers.

This book is written by and for primary healthcare teams. Its focus is on the clinical encounter, where the practitioner sees a patient or family. The primary care setting is often the first place where patients access the medical system for help with their problems. Throughout the book, we use the terms *healthcare practitioner* and *patient*. Certain sections delineate specific healthcare practitioners to illustrate how the principles apply differently according to the practitioner's time, training, and experience. We want to empower members of the primary healthcare team to feel comfortable and skilled in addressing behavioral medicine issues with patients and families.

WHAT IS BEHAVIORAL MEDICINE?

Behavioral medicine is defined as an interdisciplinary field concerned with the development and integration of behavioral, psychosocial, and biomedical knowledge and techniques relevant to the understanding of health and illness, and the application of this knowledge and these techniques to prevention, diagnosis, treatment and rehabilitation.[1,2] Behavioral medicine practitioners include physicians, social workers, nurses, midwives, and community healthcare workers working with vulnerable populations.

Behavioral medicine is at the intersection of three practice models familiar to practitioners in developing countries, namely the medical model, the public health model and the traditional medicine model. Each model has a different perspective with regard to causes and solutions related to patient problems. The medical model looks at the biological determinants of health. Its treatments include medications, surgery, diet, and other healthy lifestyle choices. The traditional medicine model has an individual focus with explanations for poor health that are rooted in a given society or group. Its beliefs about wellness and healing are often based on body balance, weather, and supernatural forces, and include treatments such as herbal remedies, acupuncture, shamanism, and cupping or coining to rid the body of negative forces or spirits. The public health model focuses on the social, economic, and

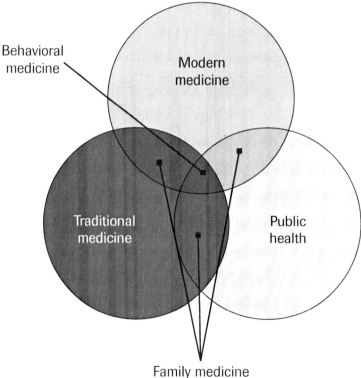

FIGURE 1.1 Behavioral medicine at the intersection of modern medicine, traditional medicine, and public health.

environmental causes of poor health. It works towards involving communities in addressing system issues that impact on health.

Figure 1.1 depicts behavioral medicine at the intersection, or the heart, of the medical, traditional medicine, and public health models of care.

Practitioners with good behavioral medicine skills successfully combine the following:

➤ assessment, diagnosis, treatment, and management skills of the medical model
➤ knowledge of community needs and resources in order to successfully apply strategies to meet the community needs of the public health model
➤ cultural beliefs and ideas about cause, cure, and treatment of traditional medicine practices.

With its basis in Western medicine, the bias of behavioral medicine is that:

1 science and reason are tools for advancing the human condition
2 if practitioners understand and use these tools, the health of their patients and communities will improve as a result.

It is important for practitioners to be aware that many people from non-Western cultures do not share this bias. The tools and strategies described in this book need to stand beside or be adapted to these differing worldviews and practices. The practitioners from these cultures are in the best position to determine what will be beneficial and how best to adapt the models and practices to their settings.

WHY INCLUDE BEHAVIORAL MEDICINE IN PRIMARY CARE?

In their book, *World Mental Health: Problems and Priorities in Low-Income Countries*, Robert Desjarlais and colleagues call attention to the impact of mental illness and behavior-induced illness on disability.[3] Figure 1.2, which was created from data reported in this book, clearly illustrates how significantly mental and behavioral health issues affect disability. It shows neuropsychiatric disorders accounting for 12% of the global burden of disease, and behavioral-related conditions accounting for 13% (vaccine-preventable illnesses, poor nutrition, and HIV/AIDS) to 32% (injuries and prenatal disorders).[4] These figures are in fact even higher when smoking and other lifestyle issues that contribute to disability are included. Certainly public health measures are needed to address many of these issues. Behavioral medicine principles are needed to help primary care practitioners to address these conditions at the point of care.

The World Health Organization (WHO) recommends that it should be primary healthcare practitioners who bring mental health and behavioral healthcare to the community level of care.[5,6] Desjarlais and colleagues suggest basic principles for countries to improve mental health services, which include the following:

➤ national and regional commitment to mental healthcare
➤ deinstitutionalization and decriminalization of mental illness
➤ development of community psychiatry
➤ development of special mental health units in district hospitals

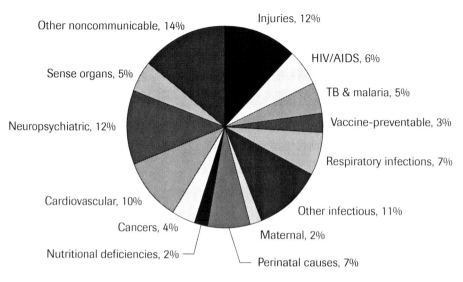

FIGURE 1.2 Disability adjusted life years (DALYs) lost, by cause. *The DALY is a health gap measure – that is, potential years of healthy life lost due to poor health or disability and premature death. It can be thought of as one less year of healthy life. Reproduced with permission from World Health Organization. Adapted from World Bank. *World Development Report 1993: investing in health*; www-wds.worldbank.org/external/default/WDSContentServer/WDSP/IB/1993/06/01/000009265_3970716142319/Rendered/PDF/multi0page.pdf (accessed 9 February 2009).

➤ the use of psychiatrists as teachers and consultants to non-physician primary practitioners
➤ the involvement of families in care and recovery
➤ the use of public health interventions (safety, clean air and water, shelter, and food) to prevent and reduce disability.[3]

Mental health disorders are among the leading causes of ill health and disability worldwide. Nearly two-thirds of individuals with known mental health disorders do not seek help from a health professional.[5] Mental health specialists need to be involved in teaching and consulting with primary care practitioners. Models exist in many parts of the developing world, where psychiatrists and other non-physician practitioners support the care provided by the primary care practitioners (*see* Chapter 10).

CORE PRINCIPLES OF BEHAVIORAL MEDICINE
Based on over 30 years of training family physicians, the Society of Teachers of Family Medicine has developed core principles to guide behavioral medicine teaching and practice. Those who apply these principles:
➤ use biopsychosocial and relationship-centered approaches to care
➤ promote patient self-efficacy and behavior change as primary factors in health promotion, disease prevention, and chronic disease management. Self-efficacy

is the belief that one has the ability to make the changes necessary to improve one's overall health

➤ integrate mental health and substance abuse care into primary healthcare services

➤ integrate psychological and behavioral knowledge into the care of physical symptoms and diseases

➤ promote the integration of sociocultural factors within the organization and delivery of healthcare services

➤ emphasize the impact of familial, social, cultural, spiritual, and environmental contexts in patient care to improve health outcomes

➤ practice a developmental and life cycle perspective with learners and clients

➤ encourage and support practitioner self-awareness, empathy, and well-being.[7]

Behavioral medicine content is well documented, but who teaches it, how it will be taught, and what priorities will be emphasized depend on a country's culture, traditions, and resources. Behavioral medicine principles and practices that are deemed important to a country or community are based on multiple factors, such as educational level of practitioners, economic conditions, and cultural norms. A 2007 survey of Vietnamese family medicine and public health faculty cited behavioral change as the top priority for the behavioral medicine curriculum, with mental health assessment and treatment being the lowest priority.[8] This may not be so unusual for developing countries, where major health improvements can be seen through changing behaviors related to sanitary practices, maternal–child nutritional habits, and childbirth delivery choices. In Vietnam and other developing countries, mental health assessment and treatment have been predominantly the responsibility of psychiatrists working in hospital settings, and not of primary healthcare practitioners.

Vietnam's family medicine and social service training systems have embraced behavioral medicine principles and have been eager to learn practical applications. In many countries this has been impossible, given the limited resources or different priorities of those in charge. Economic conditions play a major role. Vietnam's annual gross domestic product (GDP) has increased by 8–20% per year over the past two decades.[9] This strong economic growth has enabled the government to place physicians in 80% of the communal health centers, and it is now working to achieve mental health at the communal level of care. The primary goal is to have well-trained behavioral medicine teams functioning in communities to meet the needs of the population.[10]

BIOPSYCHOSOCIAL APPROACH TO CARE

A biopsychosocial approach to care is characterized by the practitioner being curious enough to assess the biological, psychological, and social factors of a patient's life, regardless of the initial complaint.[10] McDaniel and colleagues describe family-oriented healthcare as a biopsychosocial approach that recognizes that:

1   the primary focus of healthcare is the patient in the context of the family

2   the patient, family and providers are partners in healthcare

3 reflection by providers on how they are part of the treatment system is an important component of their ability to heal and care for patients.[11]

A strictly medical approach to an 8-year-old boy who comes to the doctor with abdominal pain would be to take a good medical history, check for fever, perform an abdominal examination and, depending on the findings and availability, order lab tests or an abdominal X-ray. A biopsychosocial approach would include inquiring into the context of this boy's life, beginning with the patient's ideas and reactions to his illness, and then branching out to contributing factors in the household, school, extended family, and community, and might even consider environmental influences, such as air pollution or untreated water (*see* Figure 1.3). What stresses are occurring at home or at school? What sort of relationship exists between parent and child? Does the child appear scared or depressed? Is the family

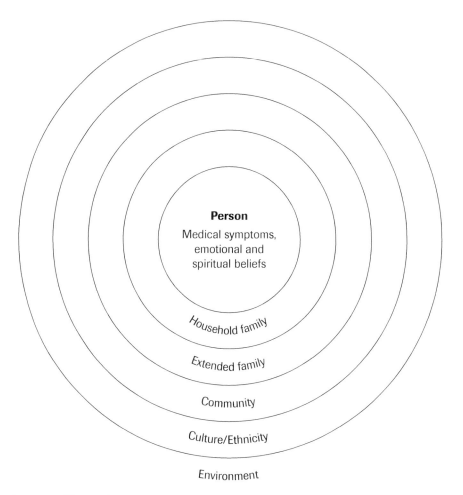

FIGURE 1.3 The psycho-social-spiritual components of the biopsychosocial model. Adapted from Engel GL. The clinical application of the biopsychosocial model. *Am J Psychiatry.* 1980; **37**: 535–44.

under a lot of stress to meet even basic needs? A practitioner could be overlooking interpersonal violence at home or at school, which medical professionals in most countries consider to be a health issue. If they focus only on the medical aspects of the case, the practitioner might not understand the true cause or factors contributing to the abdominal pain, and would thus miss the solution that would alleviate the pain.

RELATIONSHIP-CENTERED CARE

A relationship-centered approach to care holds healing relationships at the heart of humane and effective healthcare. This includes healing relationships between patients, their families, practitioners, other members of the healthcare team, and community providers. Healing relationships include empathy, compassion, and respect. A practitioner's use of good communication skills has been shown to increase patient satisfaction, adherence to treatment, physical functioning, and resolution of symptoms (including physical and emotional symptoms), and to decrease malpractice suits.[12,13] These have been shown to be malleable skills that can be taught and assessed in medical education.[14]

Yet healing is much more than the use of evidence-based psychosocial communication skills. Healing is the result of a positive relationship between the healthcare practitioner and the patient. It has the potential to transform and empower both the patient and the practitioner. The patient develops a healthier worldview or quality of life than they had when they first sought care. The practitioner develops clarity and insight about what they bring to patient care that is healing both to them and to the patient.

International consensus statements on physician–patient communication describe the essential elements of a patient-centered approach in which the physician balances the needs, wishes, and expertise of the patient with the knowledge, skills, and plan of the physician (*see* Table 2.1 in Chapter 2).[11] Consensus statements call for a planned and coherent communication curriculum for medical schools, residency training programs, and continuing physician education.[13] Recommendations state that teaching and assessment should:

➤ have a broad view of communication, including relationship skills with patients and colleagues, ethics, and the nature and context of the physician–patient relationship
➤ be consistent and compatible with patients' culture
➤ define, promote, and measure learners' ability to use a patient-centered approach to care
➤ be assessed directly with regard to how learners apply the communication tasks – for example, by using role play and directly observing or videotaping learner–patient encounters
➤ be routinely evaluated for feedback and direction
➤ foster personal and professional growth.[15]

Chapters 2 and 8 discuss this in more detail, and describe the basic communication skills to incorporate into clinical care.

BEHAVIORAL CHANGE

The impact of behavioral factors on biological health and the effectiveness of healthcare practitioners helping patients to modify unhealthy behaviors are well recognized. Approximately 50% of all causes of morbidity and mortality in the USA are linked to behavioral and social factors.[16] Worldwide, five of the ten leading causes of death fall into the categories of communicable diseases, prenatal complications, and nutritional disorders.[17] Key behavioral factors include a sedentary lifestyle, poor diet, tobacco use, alcohol consumption, psychological distress, and risky sexual behaviors.[18]

Brief interventions by healthcare practitioners have been shown to effectively improve health behaviors for a range of problems.[19,20] Prochaska and DiClemente's model of behavior change provides a way for healthcare practitioners to assess and respond to patients' attitudes and commitment to healthy change.[21] This model describes behavioral change as a process – a series of discrete phases – in which the practitioner's response is dependent on the patient's stage of change (*precontemplation, contemplation, preparation, action* or *maintenance*). It is based on a theory which states that individuals are strongly motivated to maintain a sense of autonomy and to resist coercion by others. This model recommends that practitioners relate in a way that matches the patient's stage of change, to inspire them to make the changes that are needed to improve their health. The application of this model is called *motivational interviewing*. Healthcare practitioners have successfully used motivational interviewing techniques to help patients to make behavioral changes related to the use of tobacco, drugs, alcohol, diet, and other lifestyle changes needed to improve health.

Motivational interviewing tools and techniques are available to help practitioners to modify their own unhealthy behaviors.[22,23] The rationale is that by applying these techniques to their own struggles, practitioners can better understand the struggles and successes of others, and therefore inspire others to change, regardless of the behavior. Chapter 4 discusses in detail the available tools and resources for motivational interviewing and other behavioral change strategies.

MENTAL HEALTH AND SUBSTANCE ABUSE ISSUES

There are common mental health issues that can be easily treated in primary healthcare settings. Primary care screening and treatment algorithms for mental health and substance abuse issues have been developed by the WHO and others.[24] Brief primary care interventions have been shown to be effective for substance use.[25] Early diagnosis and treatment are key to minimizing the course of the illness throughout a patient's lifetime. Early diagnosis can reduce the number of lifetime cycles of depression and schizophrenic breaks.

Mental health disorders account for 12% of the WHO global burden of disease, and constitute a larger burden than AIDS, TB, and malaria combined (10%).[26] Neuropsychiatric conditions account for up to 25% of all disability-adjusted life years (*see* Figure 1.1).[19] By the year 2020, major depression will be second only to ischemic heart disease in contributing to the loss of life years in terms of productivity and social functioning.[26] At any given moment, 10% of the general population and 20% of primary care patients will have a mental health disorder.[20] In contrast to the situation in developing countries, the US primary care system has become the de facto mental health system of the country. Approximately 50% of US patients with mental health conditions receive psychotropic medication from primary care practitioners rather than from psychiatrists.

Mental health disorders are risk factors for the development of communicable and non-communicable disease, and contribute to accidental and non-accidental injuries. Patients with chronic health conditions are two to three times more likely to have mental health and substance abuse disorders than the general population. Mental health disorders can delay help-seeking, affect adherence to treatment, increase risky behaviors, and contribute to and be compounded by chronic disease.[27]

Medication interventions for depression are as cost-effective as anti-retroviral therapy for HIV/AIDS.[28] Thus it is important for healthcare practitioners to be familiar with the identification and treatment of mental health issues in children and adults. Social workers, nurses, and other community service practitioners can counsel and support patients and families in adhering to psychotropic medication regimes, or in learning new ways of thinking and behaving to improve their health.

Several counseling approaches have been successfully applied in primary healthcare in developing counties as diverse as Afghanistan, Chile, India, and China. Interpersonal and cognitive–behavioral therapy for depression has been shown to be as effective as medication in Uganda and Pakistan.[29,30] Additional psychosocial treatments that are important for healthcare practitioners include crisis intervention, brief supportive counseling, and family counseling. These techniques are described in more detail in the chapters on family systems (*see* Chapter 5), mental health (*see* Chapter 7), and psychosocial treatments (*see* Chapter 8).

PSYCHOLOGICAL AND BEHAVIORAL CONTRIBUTIONS TO ILLNESS

Patients often present to healthcare practitioners with multiple physical concerns, which may be caused by or severely complicated by psychological, behavioral, social, or spiritual factors. Individual counseling approaches and system modifications exist to address this in primary care. A study that was conducted in an internal medicine outpatient clinic in a US hospital demonstrated that, of the top 10 symptoms presented over a 6-month period, only 16% had an established organic cause.[31] The findings of this study suggest that the practitioner should consider other causes, including the possible influence of psychological and social factors on why a patient seeks help. It is estimated that, in the USA, 30% of patients in primary care have a diagnosable mental health disorder, and 70% of patient visits are for psychosocial concerns.[32]

The concept that the mind influences the body has long been associated with traditional Eastern cultures. Numerous studies have linked internal or external stresses to decreased immune functioning. Internal stresses can include chronic medical diseases such as cardiovascular disease, diabetes, arthritis, or habits of thinking that contribute to or point to a mental health disorder.[33] External stresses can include financial pressures, the loss of a loved one, or family conflict. A stress response can even be created by what we think of as a positive stress, such as marriage, moving to a new home, or the birth of a baby.

Based on years of research with large populations, Holmes and Rahe developed a scale to measure stress in a person's life, with each stress being allocated a different score (*see* Table 1.1). Studies have validated this instrument across cultures as a way of relating stress to physical health. A cumulative score of over 300 indicates a high risk, and a score in the range 150–300 indicates a moderate risk of illness.[34] Some individuals can handle stresses without mishap. Others have difficulty coping, and even minor stresses have a negative effect on their physical, mental, or social functioning. Studies have shown that an accumulation of stresses indicated in the Holmes–Rahe Social Adjustment Scale precedes the development of a wide range of physical and emotional disorders.[34,35]

Patients often present to healthcare practitioners with physical complaints that lack an organic cause, and expect a medical cure. Chapter 3 illustrates how the patient's presentation of this type of illness can be culturally determined, and suggests strategies for addressing this type of presentation with patients, families, and other community healers.

TABLE 1.1 The Holmes–Rahe Social Adjustment Scale

Event	Stress score
Death of partner	100
Divorce	75
Marital separation	65
Jail term	63
Death of close family member	63
Personal injury or illness	53
Marriage	50
Dismissal from work	47
Marital reconciliation	45
Retirement	45
Change in health of family member	44
Pregnancy	40
Sexual difficulties	39
Gain of new family member	39
Business readjustment	39
Change in financial state	38
Death of close friend	37
Change to different line of work	36
Change in number of arguments with partner	31
Major mortgage	30
Foreclosure of mortgage or loan	29

Event	Stress score
Change in responsibilities at work	29
Son or daughter leaving home	29
Trouble with in-laws	28
Outstanding personal achievement	26
Partner begins or stops work	26
Begin or end school	25
Change in living conditions	24
Revision of personal habits	23
Trouble with boss	20
Change in working hours or conditions	19
Change in residence/schools/recreation	18
Change in social activities	17
Small mortgage or loan	16
Change in sleeping/eating habits	15
Change in number of family get-togethers	15
Vacation	13
Christmas	12
Minor violations of the law	11

Adapted with permission from Elsevier from Holmes T, Rahe R. The Social Readjustment Rating Scale. *J Psychosom Res.* 1967; **11**: 213–18.

SOCIOCULTURAL FACTORS

Medical anthropology is the study of how illnesses are perceived and treated around the world. Knowledge of anthropological models helps practitioners to develop sensitivity to patients' differing belief systems and how these systems can impede or enhance care. Practitioners can also develop awareness of their own biases and assumptions that negatively influence patient care. The models provide frameworks for interacting with patients, their families, and other members of their community.

A study of four different cultural groups in the San Francisco Bay area indicates that although patient and family reactions and disease management strategies are common, their expression differs across cultures.[36] The expression of their feelings about their disease is culturally consistent, and ranges from patients' verbal dramatization to stoic acceptance. The study also found cultural consistency in patients' perception of the extent of their illness, its impact on work and family life, and the family's influence on patients' health (*see* case scenarios in Chapter 3).

The USA is a veritable "melting pot" of different cultures. Even when patients and practitioners speak the same language, their cultures are not necessarily the same. Healthcare practitioners need to keep in mind the fact that patients may come from different cultural and ethnic backgrounds – as, for example, in the mountainous regions of Vietnam, where many ethnic groups reside in close proximity to one another. The key for practitioners is to maintain curiosity about patients' cultural background and different histories over the course of their ongoing relationship.

Care must be taken to avoid blindly believing our understandings of particular cultural groups and their influence on health. A colleague practicing in New England recently saw a 51-year-old Iraqi woman for multiple aches and pains, the most concerning of which to the patient was her stomach pain and discomfort. The patient did not speak English, routinely refused professional interpreters, and insisted on her daughter acting as her interpreter. The daughter was also a patient of the physician, and had previously expressed her concern about her mother, her prolonged period of mourning, her mother's anxieties about conditions in their homeland and the general stressors in the family. What the physician initially considered to be a condition heavily influenced by war trauma, resettlement issues, and somatic experience of distress turned out to be a heart condition. The physician was very concerned that the patient did not understand the potential risks when she refused to be immediately hospitalized for further evaluation.

It turned out that the patient was due to have an interview the following day about her immigration status. If she did not show up, she was at risk of not obtaining a residency permit, and would then not be able to return to the USA if she chose to travel. The patient refused a physician's note to reschedule the appointment, but agreed to go to the hospital immediately after her immigration appointment.

The patient did eventually come to the hospital for evaluation, her daughter remained with her throughout the stay. Her chief complaint of stomach pain was only partially resolved, and the urgent need to evaluate the cardiac condition was never understood clearly by the family, since it turned out to be a transient problem.

This case demonstrates some of the nuances and complexities in caring for people from different cultures. This practitioner's curiosity and careful listening were key to getting this patient the care that she needed. The reality for this patient was that the risks of not evaluating the heart condition were borne by her and her family in the absence of a mutually understood set of values and beliefs about the medical likelihood of her disease process, family roles, and a medical system that aims to eliminate, if at all possible, any risk of life-threatening conditions. The patient balanced out her knowledge of her symptoms with her life circumstances and made the decision not to be immediately hospitalized. Her refusal to go the hospital caused tension between the care team, the patient, and her family, but ultimately improved her overall well-being. Chapter 6 discusses more strategies and skills for providing healthcare for individuals from different cultures to our own.

THE FAMILY CONTEXT

The more practitioners know about their patients' families, the better they will be able to care for them and be a healing force in their lives. Family has both positive and negative influences on a person's health. Researchers have shown that involving the patient's partner in the care of patients with hypertension is linked to greater medication compliance, a larger decrease in blood pressure, and improvements in overall mortality.[30] Family members are more likely to share risk factors for cardiovascular disease, such as tobacco use, obesity, and high cholesterol levels.

Researchers have identified family protective factors and risk factors for health that family physicians can use to help to educate their patients.[37] Protective factors include parent coping skills, family emotional closeness, patient–family–practitioner alliance, and family time for recreation. Family risk factors include family conflict or criticism, psychological trauma related to disease and treatment, external stressors, maternal isolation, and lack of patient coping skills and disease knowledge.

The quality of family relationships also influences health. Family cohesion (either over-protection or rejection) has been linked to poor blood pressure control and poor diabetic control.[38] High levels of perceived criticism are associated with frequent use of outpatient health services.[39] Enmeshment, over-protectiveness, rigidity, and conflict avoidance have been associated with poor diabetes control among patients with type 1 diabetes and anorexia nervosa.[40] Adverse childhood experiences, including abuse, neglect, and family dysfunction, are major risk factors for multiple physical and mental illnesses, early death, and poor quality of life.[41]

The most substantial research into the family's impact on adult health has been on overall mortality, cardiovascular risk factors, the prevention of heart disease, and the course of chronic disease. Studies indicate that widowers and divorcees have higher than normal death rates.[42] Widowers who remarry have a lower death rate than others, indicating that remarriage is a protective factor. Socially isolated adults have a mortality rate that is more than twice as high as that of the least isolated group.[43]

Marital/relationship stress, including extramarital affairs, alcoholism, relationship crises, or serious ongoing marital/relationship conflict, is related to decreased survival for people with congestive heart failure and women with coronary artery disease,[44] end-stage renal disorders, and breast cancer.[45] One possible explanation is that the marriage/relationship influences emotional regulation and disease management behaviors. The results of these family studies indicate that healthcare practitioners need to be more fully aware of family issues. Chapter 5 describes how this can be accomplished.

DEVELOPMENTAL AND LIFE-CYCLE PERSPECTIVES

All patients and families go through predictable stages, with each stage involving developmental tasks that are necessary in order to move on to the next stage. A knowledge of these stages is extremely helpful to healthcare practitioners when assessing for illnesses or conditions that can inhibit patients' normal development. Most physical disabilities are evident in infancy or childhood. Around 25% of mental illnesses are evident by the age of 12 years, and 75% are evident by the age of 25 years. Early detection and treatment of physical disabilities and mental illnesses decrease the influence of the disability or illness over the course of a person's life, and increase their chances of living a full and productive life.

Families also go through predictable stages, as described in Chapter 5. Knowledge of these stages allows the practitioner to be aware of the normal stresses for each stage, to guide patients through difficult times, and to encourage additional community and family support when necessary.

PRACTITIONER WELL-BEING

Through their interactions with patients, healthcare practitioners have an impact on their body, mind, and spirit, whether they intend to or not. If practitioners are not healthy or, worse still, are unaware of their own unhealthy emotions or behaviors, they can be poor models for their patients, or may even harm their patients by what they say and how they act.

Family medicine training programs have developed processes to help physicians to increase their awareness of what physicians bring to the doctor–patient relationship. The focus of this reflective practice is on increased practitioner insight to *heal* patients, rather than on procedural skills to *treat* patients. In this context, healing is defined as being with a patient in a way that helps him or her to find and use internal and external resources to get better in as many ways as possible in mind, body, and spirit.[46]

Balint and similar discussion groups are frequently used to increase practitioner self-awareness. Groups consist of 8 to 10 practitioners, take place weekly or biweekly, and are usually led by a practitioner who has been trained in the group process. Participants present their cases with the goal of focusing on what the physician brings to the doctor–patient relationship.[47] Participants focus on how they feel and think about their patients, including the intention of their interactions, their ability to address patients' needs, and the "side-effects" or unintended consequences of their relationship. The aim is to learn how to use themselves more effectively as therapeutic instruments when addressing patients' concerns. Challenging situations that can be explored include difficult patients, dying patients, and medical mistakes.

Novack suggests four core topics to cover in a curriculum on physician self-awareness, namely challenging patient situations, how practitioners' beliefs and attitudes influence care, practitioners' feelings and emotional responses to care, and practitioner self-care.[48] Like their patients' beliefs, the beliefs of practitioners are influenced by family and cultural background, gender, socio-economic background, education, and personality (e.g. whether one is an introvert or an extrovert).

Practitioners' unrecognized feelings can distort or prohibit meaningful discussions (e.g. about issues related to death and dying) or result in over- or under-involvement with the patient (e.g. getting very involved with someone who might remind one of an ill family member). Unrecognized practitioner issues that can negatively influence the health of practitioners or the care of their patients include sadness about patients, fears about death and dying, and the impact of choosing a profession in which suffering is a constant companion. Physician self-care includes balancing personal and professional lives, preventing and managing stress, setting boundaries with patients, and time management when caring for patients.

In countries that have minimal resources to meet the medical needs of their populations, reflective practice needs to be modeled by practitioners in their day-to-day experiences with patients, practicing side by side with learners during direct patient care. Chapter 9 discusses formal and informal mechanisms to address practitioner self-awareness and well-being.

CONCLUSION

This introductory chapter provides a general overview of behavioral medicine as the clinical application of principles of psychology, anthropology, sociology, and physiology. We want all readers to understand the importance of behavioral medicine and to have the fundamental strategies, skills, and resources necessary to apply behavioral medicine so as to transform their patients, themselves, and the systems in which they work. We hope that readers will be enthused and inspired to then search out additional resources that delve into more detail on each behavioral medicine topic, in order to continue their lifelong development as healers.

KEY RESOURCES

- **Society of Behavioral Medicine:** dedicated to promoting the study of the interactions of behavior with biology and the environment, and the application of that knowledge to improve the health and well-being of individuals, families, communities and populations; www.sbm.org
- **International Society of Behavioral Medicine:** encourages the formation of national or regional organizations of behavioral medicine, encourages communication and interaction about behavioral medicine issues, stimulates research, clinical, preventive and training activities, and develops guidelines for training and research; www.isbm.info

REFERENCES

1 Society of Behavioral Medicine. *Definition of Behavioral Medicine*; www.sbm.org/about/definition.asp (accessed 17 January 2008).
2 Feldman MD, Christensen JF. *Behavioral Medicine in Primary Care: a practical guide.* Stanford, CT: Appleton & Lange; 1997.
3 Desjarlais R, Eisenberg L, Good B, *et al. World Mental Health: problems and priorities in low-income countries.* Oxford: Oxford University Press; 1995.
4 World Bank. *World Development Report 1993: investing in health*; www-wds.worldbank.org/external/default/WDSContentServer/WDSP/IB/1993/06/01/000009265_3970716142319/Rendered/PDF/multi0page.pdf (accessed 8 February 2009).
5 World Health Organization. *The World Health Report 2001. Mental health: new understanding, new hope*; www.who.int/whr2001/2001/main/en/chapter2/index.htm (accessed 2 July 2004).
6 World Health Organization. *The World Health Report 2002: reducing risks, promoting healthy life*; www.who.int/whr/2002/en/ (accessed 15 January 2008).
7 Reprinted with permission from the Society of Teachers of Family Medicine (STFM) Science GoB. *Core Principles of Behavioral Medicine*; www.stfm.org/group/behavioral.cfm (accessed 15 January 2009).
8 Schirmer JM. *Survey of Priority Behavioral Medicine Areas in Vietnam.* National Family Medicine Faculty Conference, March 2007, Hue, Vietnam.
9 Marston SA, Knox PL, Liverman DM. *World Regions in Global Context: peoples, places, and environments.* 3rd ed. Upper Saddle River, NJ: Pearson Prentice Hall; 2008.
10 Collaborative Family Health Association; www.cfha.net (accessed 26 February 2007).

11 Bayer-Fetzer Conference. Essential elements of communication in medical encounters. The Kalamazoo consensus statement. *Acad Med.* 2001; **76**: 390–3.

12 Stewart M. Effective physician–patient communication and health outcomes: a review. *Can Med Assoc J.* 1995; **152**: 1423–33.

13 Stewart MA, Brown JB, Boon H, *et al.* Evidence on patient–doctor communication. *Cancer Prev Control.* 1999; **3**: 25–30.

14 Lang F, McCord R, Harvill L, *et al.* Communication assessment using the Common Ground instrument psychometric properties. *Fam Med.* 2004; **36**: 189–98.

15 Makoul G, Schofield T. Communication teaching and assessment in medical education: an international consensus statement. *Patient Educ Couns.* 1999; **37**: 191–3.

16 McGinnis JM, Foege WH. Actual causes of death in the United States. *JAMA.* 1993; **270**: 2207–12.

17 Murray C, Lopez A (eds) *The World Health Report 2002. Reducing risks, promoting healthy life.* Geneva: World Health Organization; 2002.

18 World Health Organization. *The World Health Report 2002. Reducing risks, promoting healthy life;* www.who.int/whr/2002/en/ (accessed 18 January 2009).

19 Lopez AD, Mathers C, Ezzati M, *et al. Global Burden of Disease and Risk Factors.* Washington, DC: Oxford University Press and the World Bank; 2006.

20 World Health Organization. *The World Health Report 2001. Mental health: new understanding, new hope;* www.who.int/whr2001/2001/main/en/chapter2/index.htm (accessed 2 July 2004).

21 Prochaska JO, DiClemente CC, Norcross JC. In search of how people change: applications to addictive behavior. *Am Psychol.* 1992; **47**: 1102–14.

22 Botelho R. *Motivate Healthy Habits: stepping stones to lasting change.* New York: MHH Publications; 2004.

23 Botelho R. *Motivational Practice: promoting healthy habits and self-care of chronic diseases.* New York: MHH Publications; 2004.

24 World Health Organization. *Management of Common Mental Health Problems by General Practitioners;* www.searo.who.int/en/Section1174/Section1199/Section1630_12925.htm (accessed 3 April 2008).

25 Babor TF, Grant M, Acuda W, *et al.* A randomized clinical trial of brief interventions in primary care: summary of a WHO project. *Addiction.* 1994; **89**: 657–78.

26 World Health Organization. *The World Health Report 2001. Mental health: new understanding, new hope;* www.who.int/whr2001/2001/main/en/chapter2/index.htm (accessed 2 July 2004).

27 Prince M, Patel V, Saxena S, *et al.* No health without mental health. *Lancet.* 2008; **370**: 859–77.

28 Patel V, Aroya R, Chatterjees A, *et al.* Treatment and prevention of mental disorders in low-income and middle-income countries. *Lancet.* 2007; **370**: 991–1005.

29 Bass JK, Bolton PA, Murray LK. Do not forget culture when studying mental health. *Lancet.* 2007; **370**: 918–19.

30 Rahman A. Challenges and opportunities in developing a psychological intervention for perinatal depression in rural Pakistan – a multi-method study. *Arch Women Ment Health.* 2007; **10**: 211–19.

31 Kroenke K. Common symptoms in ambulatory care: incidence, evaluation, therapy and outcome. *Am J Med.* 1989; **86**: 262–6.

32 Strosahl K. Confessions of a behavior therapist in primary care: the odyssey and the ecstasy. *Cogn Behav Pract.* 1996; **3**: 1–28.

33 Kabat-Zinn J. *Full Catastrophe Living: using the wisdom of your body and mind to face stress, pain, and illness.* New York: Dell Publishing; 1999.

34 Holmes TH, Rahe RH. The Social Readjustment Rating Scale. *J Psychosom Res.* 1967; **11**: 213–18.

35 Cohen F. Stress and bodily illness. *Psychiatr Clin North Am*. 1981; **4**: 269–86.
36 Fisher L. *Managing chronic disease in families: similarities and differences among ethnic groups*. Families and Health Conference of the Society of Teachers of Family Medicine, 25–9 February 2004, Amelia Island, FL.
37 Weihs K, Fisher L, Baird M. Families, health, and behavior: a section of the commissioned report by the Committee on Health and Behavior: Research, Practice, and Policy Division of Neuroscience and Behavioral Health and Division of Health Promotion and Disease Prevention Institute of Medicine, National Academy of Sciences. *Fam Syst Health*. 2001; **20**: 7–46.
38 Fiscella K, Franks P, Shields CG. Perceived family criticism and primary care utilization: psychosocial and biomedical pathways. *Fam Process*. 1997; **36**: 25–41.
39 Fiscella K, Campbell TL. Association of perceived family criticism with health behaviors. *J Fam Pract*. 1999; **48**: 128–34.
40 Minuchin S, Rosman BL, Baker L. *Psychosomatic Families*. Cambridge, MA: Harvard University Press; 1978.
41 Felitti VJ, Anda RF, Nordenberg D, *et al*. The relationship of adult health status to childhood abuse and household dysfunction. *Am J Prev Med*. 1998; **14**: 245–58.
42 Kraus AS, Lillenfeld AM. Some epidemiological aspects of the high mortality rate in the young widowed group. *J Chronic Dis*. 1959; **10**: 207–17.
43 Berkman LF, Syme SL. Social networks, host resistance and mortality: a nine-year follow-up study of Alameda County residents. *Am J Epidemiol*. 1979; **109**: 186–204.
44 Weihs K, Fisher L, Baird M. *Families and the management of chronic disease*. Families and Health Conference of the Society of Teachers of Family Medicine, 23–7 February 2000, San Diego, CA.
45 Weihs K. *Marital quality: a protective factor against early death*. Families and Health Conference of the Society of Teachers of Family Medicine, 5–29 February 2004, Amelia Island, FL.
46 Waters D, Rudolph A. *A curriculum in healing*. Annual Conference of the Society of Teachers of Family Medicine, 28 February – 1 March 2001, Denver, CO.
47 Balint M. *The Doctor, his Patient and the Illness*. New York: International Universities Press; 1957.
48 Novack DH, Suchman AL, Clark W, *et al*. Calibrating the physician: personal awareness and effective patient care. *JAMA*. 1997; **278**: 502–9.

CHAPTER 2

Why behavioral medicine in primary care training?

Alain J Montegut, Pham Huy Dung and Kamlesh Bhargava

CASE SCENARIO

Noora Belushi is a 34-year-old woman living in Oman who has come to consult a primary care physician about a backache, which she has been experiencing for the past 10 months. Upon inquiry, Noora says that her backache is primarily in the lower back. It is a dull ache throughout the day and night. There is no radiation of pain to the thighs and no numbness or tingling in her legs. Over the past two weeks the backache has become more severe. In response to questions about previous treatment, she replies that she went to a traditional healer who used branding (*wasam*), which helped her for a short time. When the pain recurred, she sought the attention of a homeopath, who gave her special pills for her condition. She also took painkillers that were not successful in completely alleviating her pain. She then went to see the pharmacist, who recommended the use of a medicine which, like the others, was not helpful.

On examination, she is found to have some tenderness in the lower back, but her neurological examination is normal. The physician tells her that her exam is normal and he feels that she needs to see a specialist. Noora replies that the backache is one of a number of things that she is concerned about. The physician has many patients waiting, is in a hurry, and insists on an orthopedic referral. Noora does not want to see the orthopedic surgeon, as she will have to take a day off work and lose her daily wage. The physician tells her that that is the best he can do as he is very busy. Noora is close to tears. The physician makes a note in the patient's file that she has refused to see a specialist despite being advised to do so, and he calls in the next patient.

INTRODUCTION

This chapter reviews the pertinent history of the doctor–patient relationship in the Western medical model of care. Noora's case illustrates how practitioners can apply the biopsychosocial model to patients who are seen in primary care settings. It provides specific recommendations for an overall approach which has the potential to increase patients' satisfaction and improve clinical outcomes.[1]

Physicians encounter many influences on illnesses every day when seeing patients. However, their approach to patients can range from recognition and acceptance to ignorance or denial of these outside influences on patients. In the scenario described above, the physician's focus was quite narrow, concentrating on the biological, pathological, and scientific basis for Noora's backache. It could have been expanded to include the emotional, familial, social and cultural factors that were affecting Noora's life.

Before the early 1900s in the Western world, physicians could do little more for ill patients than come to the bedside with a small bag of herbs and liniments. They would sit with the patient and family and offer an attentive ear, a knowing nod, and a supportive hand. The most valuable therapeutic tool was the doctor's use of himself.[2] With the advances in medical knowledge and technology in the last century, physicians have acquired powerful new tools for assessing, diagnosing, and treating disease. Consequently, there has been a tendency for physicians to stay in the office, close their ears to anything other than medical information, and withdraw their hands from patients, in effect neglecting one of the most valuable tools available to the physician for healing, namely the physician himself.

We recognize that, in many parts of the world, primary healthcare practitioners might be physicians, as in Noora's case, or in countries where the primary healthcare system is not fully developed, they could more often be nurses, midwives, or health workers. For scenarios in subsequent chapters, we have made a concerted effort to vary the type of practitioner and the gender of practitioners and patients.

THE PRACTITIONER–PATIENT RELATIONSHIP

As a healthcare practitioner, do you think that Noora in the above scenario was satisfied with this encounter? If you were the practitioner, would you have been satisfied? Is there anything else about Noora that you would have wanted to know? Is there additional information that could have been helpful to this practitioner? Will Noora get better following her visit? Do you think the practitioner made an important contribution to Noora's health? Did this encounter feel satisfactory or adversarial?

Unfortunately, this is an example of a physician–patient interaction that is quite common. It did not feel particularly satisfying. It felt adversarial to both the physician and the patient. The reason for this type of interaction is heavily influenced both by the way most physicians have been trained and by the past healthcare experiences of our patients. Many physicians have been taught to view patients as "unreliable narrators". First-year medical students are taught to document patient observations in a way that hints at the mistrust in the relationship, by adding notations such as the "patient believes" or the "patient denies."[3]

Historically, for the doctor, illness has been a disease process that can be measured and understood through laboratory tests and clinical observations. The doctor's focus has been on advances in medical science and technology, not on the patient's emotions and feelings.[4] The emotional disruption is often of more concern to the patient than is the illness, and may undermine their adjustment to the disease.[5] A patient feels supported and satisfied when they feel that they have been heard and understood by the physician.[4] The typical medical encounter does not provide this sort of support.

Through their scientific training, doctors learn a tremendous amount of new information, and as they practice, they come across even more new information every day. Whether they do so consciously or not, many new physicians tend to share much of this knowledge with their patients, unless instructed to do otherwise. Physicians often feel hurried in their encounters, doing more talking than listening.[5] A recent study found that 72% of doctors interrupt their patient's opening statement after an average of 23 seconds. Patients who were allowed to state their concerns without interruption spent an average of only 6 more seconds on their office visits than patients who did not.[6]

When doctors talk too much, they cannot listen. They often ignore the patient's emotional concerns. A study of 21 doctors at an urban, university-based clinic found that when patients dropped emotional clues or talked openly about emotions, the doctor seldom acknowledged their feelings. Instead the conversation was directed back to technical talk.[7] Feedback from video-taped physician–patient encounters is an excellent method for teaching about this.

As long ago as 400 BC, Hippocrates wrote of how "the patient, though conscious that his condition is perilous, may recover his health simply through his contentment with the goodness of the physician."[8] Half a century ago physicians paid little attention when they were told that what mattered was "not only the medicine . . . or pills . . . but the way the doctor gave them to the patient – in fact the whole atmosphere in which the drug was given."[2] A more recent review on pain and the placebo effect concluded that the relationship between physicians and patients is tremendously powerful in treating pain, and that the way in which physicians address the differences between their own expectations and those of their patients may be more important than the specific treatment.[9]

What must occur between physicians and patients to enhance healing? Hippocrates wrote that if physicians knew nothing about their patients' lives, healing could not take place.[10] The physician must use the factors that intersect all medical, alternative, and psychological therapies in their interactions – attention, bedside manner, empathy, positive regard, compassion, hope, and enthusiasm.

THE FAMILY DOCTOR AS A UNIQUE PRIMARY CARE PHYSICIAN

Recognition that a problem exists in the patient–doctor relationship, and that physicians can do a better job of healing their patients, has led to a change in the approach to the teaching of this sacred relationship over the last half century. Now the preferred physician is the one who not only has a significant mastery of medical knowledge, but also can relate to patients in a way that allows for more satisfaction and better health. From these new criteria has emerged the development of family medicine as a new primary care discipline, with a unique body of knowledge and an educational curriculum that emphasizes the doctor–patient relationship, and care that encompasses the entire patient context.

> Family physicians possess unique attitudes, skills, and knowledge, which qualifies them to provide continuing and comprehensive medical care, health maintenance and preventive services to each member of the family regardless of sex, age, or type of problem; be it biological, behavioral, or social. These specialists, because of their background and interactions with the family, are best qualified to serve as each patient's advocate in all health-related matters, including the appropriate use of consultants, health services, and community resources.[11]

This underscores the approach that family physicians take in patient care. In addition to having a sound base of medical knowledge, family physicians look at patients with reference to the biopsychosocial model of healthcare.[12] Many countries are adopting family medicine as the specialty of choice for the delivery of primary care.[13] Training of primary care physicians benefits from the biopsychosocial behavioral science curriculum that is integral to family medicine training worldwide.[14]

THE BIOPSYCHOSOCIAL MODEL

The biopsychosocial model of medicine, in contrast to the biomedical model, is a way of looking at mind, body, and patient contexts as important and interlinked systems. If we look at our case study, we note that the physician focused only on the medical issues. There is so much more that this physician could have learned if he had included some questions about the patient's family and any social issues facing the patient.

The biopsychosocial model treats the biological, psychological, and social issues as systems of the body, similar to the traditional medical systems such as the respiratory and cardiovascular systems. A key axiom in medical anthropology is that a dichotomy exists between two aspects of sickness – disease and illness. *Disease* refers to a malfunctioning of biological and/or psychological processes, whereas the term *illness* refers to the psychosocial experience and meaning of perceived disease.[15]

The biopsychosocial model gives great importance to the illness, with physicians gathering much more information than the straightforward biological signs, symptoms, or disease processes. Using this approach, the physician inquires about the patient's psychological state, feelings and beliefs about their illness, and their expectations for each visit. The patient develops a degree of comfort and trust in their physician and is open to their inquiries about social factors which may influence their health, such as their relationship with their family and the community (*see* Figure 1.2 in Chapter 1).

> If the physician had used this type of inquiry with Noora, he would have discovered that she is a mother of five children (two boys and three girls), between the ages of 2 and 10 years. She was divorced from her husband one year ago. She is not

educated. To support her family she is working as a cleaner in a private company and is on daily wages, getting paid only for the hours that she works. Her supervisor is not supportive. Noora often has to take leave without pay because of her backache and because of the health needs of her daughter, who has sickle-cell anemia and has had frequent hospitalizations. Noora is under a lot of pressure both at home and at work, and has no family support. She has no friends, as all of her time is spent either working or doing household chores. She bought a car with a loan from the bank and is finding it difficult to pay the installments. Noora thinks that her backache is related to her physical and mental stress. She would like the doctor to confirm this belief. She also keeps changing doctors and clinics in her search for understanding, for reassurance that the backache is not cancer, and for a possible cure.

Many topics and issues can be difficult for physicians and patients to discuss. There are several ways in which physicians can bridge this gap. First, they can explore not only the patient's physical symptoms, but also the emotional effects of the symptoms on their patient. The value of patient-centered care has become an important tenet in medicine. Care that is truly patient-centered considers patients' cultural traditions, their personal preferences and values, their family situation, and their lifestyle.[16]

This patient-centered approach generally involves beginning with open-ended questions, which require a narrative response. This allows patients to talk about their illness experience in their own words, providing insight into their values and their beliefs about causes and possible cures. The physician can then move on to asking closed-ended questions, which require a yes, no or multiple choice response, to narrow down the focus. Some have called this the "funnel approach" to patient interviewing. In this way, patients become involved in the assessment and treatment of their disease, and the physician is more likely to understand how to treat their disease.

Patient-centered care is a change from a more traditional approach to the patient interview. In the latter approach, physician interviewing places the patient in a very passive position, where they are given information and direction from the physicians, with little attention being paid to the patient's concerns. Based on the research described in Chapter 1, family physicians are now taught to engage in a relationship with the patient in order to better understand their needs and feelings.

Another way in which primary care physicians can explore the emotional and social issues affecting health is through the establishment of a longitudinal relationship with the patient and their family.[17] This longitudinal relationship contributes to continuity of care and the development of trust, which are important foundations of family medicine.[18]

Through multiple encounters over a period of time, the relationship can grow, allowing trust to develop between the physician and the patient, particularly if there have been successes. This allows for ever more openness and understanding. The history of patients within the context of their families and communities can be very helpful to understanding the nature of their illnesses and what is needed for treatment and healing. Perhaps if Noora's physician had known her over a period of time and had asked and then listened to her, he would have been better able to help her with her backache.

Several questions about illness are fundamental to understanding the deductive work of the physician. Where is the illness occurring? What does the physician know about the patient's social context? Is the patient from an underserved community or an alienated ethnic group, or living on wages so low that her family's basic needs are not being met? Has the patient experienced a recent loss or trauma? In which primary sphere of influence does the symptom reside – the biological sphere, the psychological sphere, or the social sphere? Could the symptom be related to all three spheres simultaneously?

These are the sorts of questions that generalist physicians have asked themselves for generations. How can physicians gain the experience to even begin to contemplate these issues? Family medicine finds itself at the center of the nucleus of the three spheres of illness. Two of the spheres of illness can be framed within the context of the family – the biological and the emotional (or psychological) spheres. One definition of family is "any group of people related by blood or choice, who move together through time."[19] It is within families that most individuals experience their health problems.[20] Family members provide most of the healthcare in the world, and most beliefs about health are developed within the family network.[21]

The social sphere is found within the context of the community and the relationships that patients and their families have with the community. It is essential that physicians recognize this context. Physicians must be capable of applying epidemiological studies and social interventions to the clinical care of individual patients and their families. By doing so, the primary care practice itself becomes a community medicine program (*see* Chapter 6). The individual patient, their family, and the community are the foci of diagnosis, treatment, and ongoing surveillance.[22] Together they create the social context within which physicians can better understand their patients.

The patient within her social sphere is the representation through which the family physician regards behavioral medicine and its importance in enabling the delivery of high-quality and affordable healthcare. The doctor must be mindful of the patient within the three spheres of illness that allow him to practice with a biopsychosocial approach to the patient. It is within the context of family medicine that focuses on all three spheres that the physician can best integrate these concepts into the practice of medicine.

USING THE MODEL IN PATIENT ENCOUNTERS

Evidence shows that the biopsychosocial model and patient-centered care can be taught and applied in primary care settings.[23] Table 2.1 illustrates the main points of the Kalamazoo Consensus Statement, which was developed by physician trainers from throughout the world. This statement delineates the essential elements of doctor–patient communication. The elements are considered to represent the core psychosocial treatment strategy of primary care.

TABLE 2.1 Essential elements of physician–patient communication

Essential element	Tasks
Establishes rapport	• Encourages a partnership between physician and patient
	• Respects patient's active participation in decision making
Opens discussion	• Allows patient to complete opening statement
	• Elicits patient's full set of concerns
	• Establishes and maintains a personal connection
Gathers information	• Uses open- and closed-ended questions appropriately
	• Structures, clarifies, and summarizes information
	• Listens actively using non-verbal (e.g. eye contact, body position) and verbal (e.g. words of encouragement) techniques
Understands patient's perspective of illness	• Explores contextual factors (e.g. family, culture, gender, age, socio-economic status, spirituality)
	• Explores beliefs, concerns, and expectations about health and illness
	• Acknowledges and responds to patient's ideas, feelings, and values
Shares information	• Uses language that patient can understand
	• Checks for understanding
	• Encourages questions
Reaches agreement on problems and plans	• Encourages patient to participate in decision making to the extent patient desires
	• Checks patient's willingness and ability to follow the plan
	• Identifies and enlists resources and supports
Provides closure	• Asks whether patient has other issues or concerns
	• Summarizes and affirms agreement with the plan of action
	• Discusses follow-up (e.g. next visit, plan for unexpected outcomes)

Adapted from Makoul G. Essential elements of communication in medical encounters: the Kalamazoo consensus statement. *Acad Med.* 2001; **76:** 390–3.

These tasks are seen as a challenge in resource-poor countries, where annual, preventative exams may not be provided for the majority of people, and where medical practitioners may spend only 3 to 8 minutes per patient. In a continuity relationship, where patients have multiple visits over a period of time, elements such as exploring the patient's perspective may be incorporated over a series of visits and comprehensively applied in more prolonged visits such as annual exams. Simple strategies that physicians can follow to incorporate elemental concepts in their practice of medicine are described below.

1 **Establishing the relationship:** Cultivate a patient-centered partnership by encouraging and actively listening to the patient as they tell their illness story in their own words.[24] Solicit the patient's concerns and opinions by asking open-ended questions during the medical interview – for example, "What has been happening since you were here last?", "What do you think is causing

these symptoms?" or "What troubles you most about this?" Patients want to be seen as human beings, not merely as a symptom or disease category.[25] In a videotaped study of 171 office visits, it was demonstrated that doctors who encouraged patients to talk about psychosocial issues, such as their family and job, had more satisfied patients, and visits averaged only 2 minutes longer than those in which doctors had not encouraged this type of conversation.[26]

2 **Setting the agenda:** Elicit the patient's agenda for each visit. Patients and physicians often approach an encounter with different agendas. For example, the physician's agenda may be to try to identify osteoarthritis as the reason for the patient's back pain. The patient might come to the appointment believing that she has cancer and needs to see a specialist. Therefore it is important for both physician and patient to communicate their agendas at the beginning of the appointment. Physicians can best promote this by asking questions such as "What can I do for you today?", "How can I be of most help to you at this time?" or "What do you think is going on?" Eliciting all of the patient's agenda items first and then negotiating what can and cannot be dealt with can help to meet patient expectations, and can also prevent "Oh, by the way . . ." topics at the end of the encounter.

3 **Relationship building:** Work on developing a relationship of mutual trust with the patient. There are four key elements in developing trust: 1. good communication that restates goals and demonstrates interest; 2. active listening by acknowledging what you hear, seeking more information, and checking feelings; 3. using body language such as appropriate facial expressions and gestures; and 4. interactions that allow the other person to participate.[27] The health of the doctor–patient relationship is the best predictor of whether or not the patient will follow the doctor's instructions and advice. Certainly if patients follow their physician's guidance, there will probably be an improved health outcome. In the above scenario, Noora might have been more willing to divulge more personal information and participate more fully if the doctor had used simple body language that indicated his willingness to listen.

4 **Patient empowerment:** Consider the patient to be the expert on their experience of their illness.[28] The patient's knowledge and perspective of their illness is just as important to patient outcomes as is their doctor's scientific knowledge and perspective. Questions to ask patients could include "What are your ideas about the cause or cure for this symptom?" or "How is this affecting you and your family?" or "What are you hoping to get out of this visit?"[3]

5 **Establish empathy:** Be overtly empathetic by acknowledging the difficulty that the patient experiences in trying to manage their illness as they struggle to maintain their roles within family and community. In a series of reports by the Association of American Medical Colleges on the Medical School Objectives Project, it was stated that medical schools are expected to educate altruistic physicians who "must be compassionate and empathetic in caring for patients." Physicians' understanding of a patient's perspective – and their expression of caring, concern, and empathy – are among the listed educational objectives.[29] Empathy in patient-care situations is a cognitive attribute that calls for the ability to understand the patient's inner experiences and perspective, as well as the

ability to communicate this understanding. Empathy means demonstrating an understanding of the patient's pain and distress while maintaining an objective and observant stance. This is most likely to be accomplished when physicians have established longitudinal relationships with their patients and recognize the psychosocial spheres that are prevalent in their patients' lives.

6 **Cognitive concept:** Find common ground between the physician's perspective of disease and the patient's views of their illness. Physicians can educate patients about their disease, and patients can educate physicians about their illness experiences. Education plays a very important role in a good doctor–patient relationship. Education involves a dialog through which the physician elicits the patient's thoughts, feelings, and beliefs (understanding the patient's perspective), and then provides new information consistent with the patient's needs and interest. It is an important skill to present medical information in logical, basic terms in the language of the patient rather than that of the practitioner. Providing written materials enhances the information that is obtained from the physician during the appointment, but this can only be successful if the element of trust is present.[30]

Armed with this information, would we now approach our patient Noora, from the initial case study, any differently? What other questions would we ask? Would we leave her as she began to cry? Would we know how to transform the conversation to one of healing? If we asked her what her hopes were for the visit, she might have answered that she wanted medication to ease the pain and to help her sleep at night. She might also have told us that she wanted understanding and reassurance that it was nothing serious. She has trust in us and values her relationship with us, given that we have taken care of her multiple health issues since she arrived in the country. Although this was not the case for Noora, the patient could have an underlying mental health disorder that is affecting her ability to function.

In 2001, the World Health Organization (WHO) published a report on mental health.[31] A leading recommendation of this report was to integrate the assessment and treatment of mental health disorders into primary healthcare (*see* Chapter 7). This recommendation was repeated in a recent joint report by the WHO and Wonca.[32] Through the practice of patient-centered care and the use of the biopsychosocial model of care, primary care practitioners can increase their ability to identify mental health and behavioral health issues early in the course of treatment, and thus can have an impact on their patients' views of their illness and the outcomes of their disease. Physicians must certainly be aware of the biological causes of disease, but must also exhibit curiosity about the behavioral, emotional, and social issues of their patients' lives.

CONCLUSION

The discipline of family medicine has made a commitment to teach the biopsychosocial model of healthcare in its training programs. This model allows for more appropriate healthcare in assessing and providing care within the whole context of patients' lives. It allows for greater patient satisfaction in the patient–physician relationship, higher levels of adherence to treatment, and greater satisfaction of physicians in their work. We recommend widespread adoption of this model for the training and retraining of primary care physicians.

KEY RESOURCES

● *Integrating Mental Health into Primary Care: a global perspective*; www. who.int/mental_health/policy/Mental%20health%20+%20primary%20 care-%20final%20low-res%20140908.pdf (accessed 2 October 2008).
● *Integrated Primary Care: combining behavioral health and primary care:* provides resources, evidence, and training programs to integrate behavioral health into primary care; www.integratedprimarycare.com (accessed 15 April 2009).

REFERENCES

 1 Commonwealth Fund. *Patient-Centered Care*; www.commonwealthfund.org/topics/ topics_list.htm?attrib_id=15313 (accessed 21 July 2008).
 2 Balint M. *The Doctor, His Patient, and the Illness*. 2nd ed. Edinburgh: Churchill Livingstone; 1957 (reprinted 1986).
 3 Toombs K. *The Meaning of Illness: a phenomenological account of the different perspectives of physician and patient*. New York: Kluwer Academic Publishers; 1992.
 4 Roter DL, Hall JA. *Doctors Talking with Patients/Patients Talking with Doctors: improving communication in medical visits*. Westport, CT: Auburn House; 1992.
 5 Korsch BM, Harding C. *The Intelligent Patient's Guide to the Doctor–Patient Relationship*. Oxford: Oxford University Press; 1998.
 6 Marvel MK, Epstein RM, Flowers K, *et al.* Soliciting the patient's agenda: have we improved? *JAMA.* 1999; **281**: 283–7.
 7 Suchman AL, Markakis K, Beckman HB, *et al.* A model of empathic communication in the medical interview. *JAMA.* 1997; **277**: 678–82.
 8 Hojat M. *Empathy in Patient Care: antecedents, development, measurement, and outcomes*. New York: Springer-Verlag; 2007.
 9 Turner JA, Deyo RA, Loeser JD, *et al.* The importance of placebo effects in pain treatment and research. *JAMA.* 1994; **25**: 1609–14.
10 Hojat M, Gonnella JS, Nasca TJ, *et al.* Physician empathy: definition, components, measurement, and relationship to gender and specialty. *Am J Psychiatry.* 2002; **159**: 1563–9.
11 American Academy of Family Physicians. *Family Physicians' Scope of Practice*; www. aafp.org/online/en/home/policy/state/issues/scope/fpscope.html (accessed 15 January 2009).
12 Engel GL. The need for a new medical model. *Science.* 1977; **196**: 129–36.
13 Wonca. *Proceedings of the World Council Meeting, Singapore, 17–25 July 2007*. Global Family Doctor, Wonca, 2007.
14 Schirmer JM, Cartwright C, Montegut AJ, *et al.* Collaborative needs assessment and work plan in behavioral medicine curriculum development in Vietnam. *Fam Syst Health.* 2004; **22**: 410–18.
15 Kleinman A. *Patients and Healers in the Context of Culture*. Berkeley, CA: University of California Press; 1981.
16 Institute for Healthcare Improvement; www.ihi.org/IHI (accessed 21 July 2008).
17 Wissow LS, Larson SM, Roter DL, *et al.* for the SAFE Home Project. Longitudinal care

improves disclosure of psychosocial information. *Arch Pediatr Adolesc Med*. 2003; **157**: 419–24.

18 Shahady EJ. Principles of family medicine: an overview. In: Sloane P, Slatt L, Curtis P (eds) *Essentials of Family Medicine*. 2nd ed. Baltimore, MD: Williams and Wilkins; 1993. pp. 3–8.

19 McDaniel S, Campbell T, Hepworth J, *et al. Family-Oriented Primary Care*. 2nd ed. New York: Springer; 2005.

20 Campbell TL. The family's impact on health: a critical review and annotated bibliography. *Fam Syst Med*. 1986; **4**: 135–328.

21 Dougherty WA, Baird M. *Families and Health*. Beverly Hills, CA: Sage; 1988.

22 Connors KM. *An Overview of Community-Oriented Primary Care*; http://depts. washington.edu/ccph/pdf_files/handout1.pdf (accessed 16 January 2009).

23 Lang F, Floyd M, Beine K, *et al. Reaching Common Ground: core communication skills of a patient-centered clinical interview*. Johnson City, TN: Department of Family Medicine, East Tennessee State University; 1998.

24 Meland E. *Patient-Centered Method and Self-Directed Behavior Change*; www.uib.no/ isf/people/doc/eivind/thesis00.htm (accessed 18 May 2009).

25 Lown B. *The Lost Art of Healing*. Boston, MA: Houghton Mifflin Company; 1996.

26 Marvel K, Dougherty WA, Baird M. Levels of physician involvement with psychosocial concerns of individual patients: a developmental model. *Fam Med*. 1993; **25**: 337–42.

27 Lesmeister MK. *Working with Others: developing trust and cooperation*. http://edis. ifas.ufl.edu/pdffiles/FY/FY74800.pdf (accessed 16 January 2009).

28 Roter DL, Hall JA. *Doctors Talking with Patients/Patients Talking with Doctors: improving communication in medical visits*. Boston, MA: Auburn House; 1992.

29 Association of American Medical Colleges. *Medical School Objectives Project: learning objectives for medical school education*; https://services.aamc.org/Publications/showfile. cfm?file=version87.pdf&prd_id=198&prv_id=239&pdf_id=87 (accessed 18 May 2009).

30 Drossman D. *Inside the Minds: the art and science of gastroenterology*. Boston, MA: Aspatore Books: A Thomson Business; 2007.

31 World Health Organization. *The World Health Report 2001. Mental health: new understanding, new hope*; www.who.int/whr2001/2001/main/en/chapter2/index.htm (accessed 2 July 2004).

32 Funk M, Ivbajaro G (eds) *WHO/Wonca Joint Report: integrating mental health into primary care – a global perspective*. Geneva: World Health Organization; 2008.

CHAPTER 3

The mind–body connection: patients with somatic complaints with no organic cause

Julie M Schirmer and Au Bich Thuy

CASE SCENARIO 1

Marguerite is a 34-year-old Mexican woman, who has been brought by her sister to see her doctor after two days of uncontrollable pain. The day before, the patient had been in the public market when she suddenly became dizzy and collapsed on to the ground. She had been moaning in pain ever since, not eating, not sleeping, and not taking any fluids. Her family is very concerned. On exam, there are no significant findings with regard to the cause. She is sent to the hospital to address her dehydration.

CASE SCENARIO 2

Chun-Hua is a 19-year-old Chinese woman who comes with her mother to see a doctor about chronic stomach upset, which has been ongoing for the past two years, and worsening over the past six months. She describes the stomach ache as contributing to problems with sleep, fatigue, concentration, and pursuing her studies. She is one year out of high school and is studying for the medical school entry examination. She is convinced that she has cancer.

INTRODUCTION

This chapter describes culture-specific aspects of the healthcare practitioner–patient relationship, illness, disease, and the health system. It describes cognitive and behavioral counseling models for practitioners to use to help patients to deal with emotions that are interfering with their health. It also provides clues as to how practitioners can become healers who work towards curing rather than merely treating their patients' illnesses. Practitioners have little chance of curing if they deny, criticize, or refute patients' perspectives and the experiences that contribute to their illnesses.

Our bodies, minds, and emotions are intricately connected and are influenced by the cultures in which we live. Unique cultural explanations for illness, healing, and wellness are rooted in very profound observations. They are, in a sense, metaphors that have evolved over multiple generations. We may never understand them completely, but we must deeply respect them and learn to complement patients' metaphors and their culturally specific healing traditions with our care.

Both of the above cases demonstrate how culture influences the thought processes of patients, their reactions to stress, and their health-seeking behaviors. How can a healthcare practitioner best help patients to understand this mind–body connection, and help them to feel better now and in the future?

CULTURE-BOUND SYNDROMES

The above two case scenarios are examples of what are known as *culture-bound syndromes*. Culture-bound syndromes are physical symptoms with a prescribed psychiatric component that presents in idiosyncratic ways particular to a culture or geographical region. They challenge the medical model bias that symptoms are biomedical until proven otherwise.

For simplicity's sake, we refer to the medical model in this chapter as the model taught and practiced by Western-trained healthcare practitioners, who have been trained in the use of the *International Classification of Diseases, 10th Revision (ICD-10)*[1] and the *Diagnostic and Statistical Manual of Mental Disorders, Fourth Edition, Text Revision (DSM-IV-TR)*[2] to diagnose and treat physical and mental diseases. To have any chance of curing these and other culture-bound syndromes, healthcare practitioners must consider the patient's perspective, family issues, and other psychosocial issues that may be causing or contributing to their presenting symptoms.

The first scenario is typical of *ataque de nervios*, a condition commonly found in Latin American countries.[3] The ataque is similar to a prolonged panic attack with physical ramifications. It can include feeling out of control, crying, trembling, amnesia, verbal or physical aggression, and uncontrollable shouting. It is associated with stress within the family and is considered by many to be a physical manifestation of "soul trauma."

What is Marguerite's explanation or her family's explanation for the cause and treatment of her illness? What have been her life experiences up until now? What is going to make the most sense culturally to help this woman? In this case, the healthcare practitioner discovers that Marguerite's husband had been unfaithful. Marguerite had gone to the market to confront the "other woman", who worked as a flower vendor. When the mistress rebuffed her, Marguerite began to yell and scream, and eventually collapsed on the street. Her family was called to take her home. She then immediately went to bed, refusing to take any food or drink.

The healthcare practitioner easily obtained this story during the office visit, as this occurred in a culture where the demonstration of intense emotions and talk about family stress are commonplace. But how would this play out in a culture where it is not customary to talk about such issues or emotions outside the family, as is the case in the second scenario?

The second scenario takes place in China and is typical of *shenjing shuairou* or neurasthenia, commonly seen in Asian countries, where physical diagnoses are much more acceptable than psychological causes of functional impairment.[4] It is described as a decrease in vital energy (*qi*). The *Chinese Classification of Mental Disorders (CCMD-2)* states that three of the following five symptoms are required: weakness, emotional disturbance, excitement, tension-induced pain, and sleep disturbance.[5] This disorder overlaps with the Western medical diagnoses of somatization disorder, depression, anxiety, and chronic fatigue syndrome.

Prior to seeing her doctor, Chun-Hua had taken remedies that had been passed down for generations within her family. Her sister had used massage to help to alleviate the pain and discomfort. When that didn't work, she went to the acupuncturist, who burned cones of dried herbs on key points on her body (*moxa*). She eventually went to the drug store and took what the pharmacist suggested. When that also failed to work, she sought help from a doctor at a private clinic. She proceeded to get an ultrasound scan, which revealed nothing. Ultrasound scans are used frequently, regardless of the complaint. They are plentiful in many communities in the developing world, as multiple donors have provided second-hand machines.

If Chun-Hua had lived in an isolated rural community, she might have visited a herbalist (for a stronger concoction), a traditional medicine physician (for a diagnosis related to the seven organ systems), a Buddhist priest (for cleansing rituals), or a fortune teller (to perform a ceremony to rid her of evil spirits). In many countries, such as Vietnam, the government discourages many of these practices, yet the practices continue to take place in the more isolated regions of the country. The values, beliefs, and treatments of these alternative practitioners may be in harmony with how the patient and their family view the illness. If the practitioner can be sure that she is operating within the confines of the law, it is best for her to collaborate with these healers. In the above scenario, if the healthcare practitioner had ignored this previous treatment and Chun-Hua's other life circumstances, she would have missed the opportunity to fully understand her patient's beliefs and to detect possible clues to an effective treatment.

The health-seeking behaviors that are shown in this second case demonstrate that there is more to a healthcare system than the doctor, the patient, and the medical staff. Often, indigenous healers influence the patient's explanations of their symptoms as well as treatment options. This healthcare practitioner may not have incorporated other tried and tested remedies or causal explanations in her history. If she had inquired into Chun-Hua's underlying values, beliefs, and stressors, she would have increased her chances of healing (as opposed to merely treating) this patient.

THE RELAXATION RESPONSE

Over the past 50 years, researchers have linked the body's physical state to stresses in the psychosocial spheres. Hans Selye initially proposed the concept of a stress response as the body's natural reaction to help to mobilize resources when threatened.[6] The stress response has been described as the "fight or flight response", triggering hormones in order either to prepare to confront danger, or to escape from danger. In short bursts, the stress response can be life-saving. However, in the long term it can damage the body by exacerbating pain, chronic disease, and mental health conditions. Chronic exposure to the stress hormones can cause cumulative strain on several organs and tissues, but especially on the cardiovascular system. These physiological symptoms provide the incentive to learn how to respond to stress in healthier ways.

Many cultures are oriented towards giving attention to physical pain but not to emotional pain. With regard to emotional pain, healthcare practitioners can use brief behavioral therapy for anxiety symptoms, and cognitive therapy for symptoms of depression, anxiety, and physical or emotional pain. Every physical symptom has medical, psychological, and psychosocial components. Healthcare practitioners need to be aware of all three components.

Healthcare practitioners can educate patients about the physiological causes of panic attacks and *ataques de nervios*. Perceived stress causes an increase in the release of adrenaline, which leads to hyperventilation, shortness of breath, dizziness, skin temperature changes, and the sudden awareness of one's heartheart. As with Marguerite, many people who experience panic believe that they are dying, going mad, or having a heart attack. A physician can rule out a heart condition or other medical conditions, and can discuss the benign nature of panic. He or other primary care staff can then explain and demonstrate deep breathing techniques to patients (behavioral therapy), and follow up over the course of several visits. Deep breathing involves taking slow, deep inward breaths on a count of four, holding on a count of four, and slowly breathing out on a count of four. Another model uses counts of four, seven, and eight, respectively.

Herbert Benson, a Harvard cardiologist, became interested in researching the *relaxation response*, which is a physiological state that is in direct contrast to the stress response.[7] The relaxation response has long existed in religious teachings. It can be produced in a variety of ways, from meditation and visualization to yoga, exercise, or listening to calming music or sounds. It can be elicited by:

1 sitting or lying in a comfortable position with the eyes closed or focused on a distant point on the wall or ground
2 focusing on a word or phrase
3 noticing and letting go of other thoughts that come into one's awareness.

Practicing the relaxation response produces multiple positive effects on the body, such as decreasing the heart rate and blood pressure. Breathing rate and oxygen consumption also decline, blood flow to the muscles decreases, and blood flow to the brain and skin increases, producing a feeling of warmth and rested mental alertness.[8] Daily practice of the relaxation response, even for just five minutes, can alleviate common mental illnesses and stress-related medical conditions.

COGNITIVE THERAPY

Aaron Beck, a highly respected US psychiatrist, developed a cognitive therapy model that portrays a person's mind as the interpreter of external and internal stressors and as the mediator between perceived stress and the body's response to stress. People with depression, anxiety, multiple somatic complaints, and chronic pain are likely to have developed health-defeating habits of thinking that worsen their illnesses and disabilities. These negative habits of thinking, or *cognitive distortions*, can be modified or even replaced by thoughts that contribute to health, happiness, and well-being.

Most of us can identify with some of the unhealthy thoughts described in Table 3.1. It is the constant use of them that has a negative impact on one's mental and physical health. Counseling involves education about the effects of cognitive distortions on the body and the mind, along with skills to identify, label, and reframe the cognitive distortions.

TABLE 3.1 List of health-defeating thoughts

Helplessness	You feel that you have no control over your life. You think that nothing that you do will make a difference
All good/all bad dichotomy	You see people, situations, or events as either all good or all bad
Self-criticism	You feel that if you make a mistake, then you are bad, incompetent, or "a loser"
Pessimism	You think that if anything could possibly go wrong, it will
Absolute thinking	You feel that you or others must, should, ought to or need to act, speak, or think in an infallible and specific way
Owning the problem	You feel that you own a specific unhealthy condition ("I am depressed. I always have been depressed and I always will be depressed")
Unlucky thinking	You feel that you are unlucky and that bad things will always happen to you
"Yes but . . ." thinking	You refuse to make any changes that might improve your health, and you come up with barriers and multiple reasons why you cannot consider changing ("That's just the way I am")
Comparing	You judge yourself predominantly on the basis of what others have, not what you have

Cognitive therapy helps patients to transform health-defeating thoughts into health-promoting thoughts. This type of therapy may not work so easily with patients who are not accustomed to discussing the intimate details of their thoughts and emotions with medical practitioners, as in the case of Chun-Hua. Practitioners can use the concepts of motivational interviewing (*see* Chapter 4) to move patients to an emotional state of mind which will make them more open to discussing these issues with healthcare practitioners. They can take the following steps to help patients when their negative habits of thinking are interfering with their health:

1 **Educate patients** about how their mind affects their body and their emotions, and how it is possible to change how they think in order to change how they feel. As Chun-Hua talked about her thoughts and her reactions to her physical symptoms, she revealed fears of not passing her exams, and of failing herself and her parents.

2 **Identify patients' negative statements** when they occur during the office visit. A list of common health-defeating thought patterns can help healthcare practitioners in this process. Chun-Hua repeatedly told herself "I'm such a loser. I'll never be able to pass this test."

3 **Help to reframe the unhealthy statements.** Is the negative thought really true? What is a more reasonable and health-promoting thought, as opposed to a health-defeating thought? This might be as far as the doctor gets. A nurse or community health worker could use worksheets[9] or lists of reframing statements to continue the counseling process (*see* Table 3.2 for an example of reframing in a Muslim context).[10] Chun-Hua had been in the top 10% of her class and had always excelled academically. Her anxiety had helped her to study in the past, but now it was overwhelming her. The practitioner helped her to acknowledge that she hadn't failed before, that she was a very hard worker, and that her hard work most often met with success.

TABLE 3.2 Cognitive reframing statements modified with Islamic tenets

Increasing ability to change	*Allah* (God) gave us free will, including the ability to control our *naif* (self). Allah has given us many opportunities to practice self-control through fasting during Ramadan and weekly *sunna* (traditional fasting). These are ways, with the help of Allah, in which we can enhance our self-discipline and change for the better
Addressing all good/all bad thinking	We have worth because we are created by Allah. We are created with strengths and weaknesses
Addressing self-criticism and developing a high frustration tolerance	Misfortunes and blessings are from Allah. Misfortunes are not terrible or awful, but rather a test. Although adversities may be unpleasant, we can withstand them. Allah tells us that He will not test us beyond what we can bear. By reminding ourselves of Allah's goodness, and engaging in regular *dua* (informal prayer), we can cope with life's challenges
Accepting others	Because people are created with weaknesses, they will make mistakes. Islam tells us not to judge others for their shortcomings, but to accept people with their strengths and weaknesses
Accepting oneself	Although human approval and accomplishment are beneficial, they are not necessary for a productive life. As it says in the Qu'ran, for him who relies on Allah, Allah is enough for him
Developing love of self	Although it is nice to have the favor of others, we do not need the approval of others. True satisfaction and solace are found in our relationship with Allah. Our regular remembrance of Allah helps us to know that He loves us

Accepting responsibility	Although facing difficulties is often challenging, Islam reminds us to persevere through adversity. No one else will bear our burdens for us. Each of us is responsible for our actions and the paths that we choose
Accepting self-direction	Allah has blessed us with His *risz* (provisions/resources). Consequently, we are not dependent on others for our needs. Rather, we strive for *tawakil* (reliance on Allah for all our needs)
Self-acceptance	Allah knows us better than we know ourselves. Allah knows our weaknesses. Allah knows we make mistakes. Consequently, we can take comfort in Allah's mercy and accept ourselves with our strengths and weaknesses

4 **Affirm that habits of thinking can be changed.** In the same way that we learn a new language or a musical instrument, with education and practice people can change habits of thinking to improve their quality of life and how they feel. The more a person practices, the more quickly they can master the change in thinking.

5 **Refer to and collaborate** with other team members, community providers, or printed resources. The World Health Organization, the World Federation for Mental Health, and others have excellent handouts translated in multiple languages to help practitioners and patients through the cognitive therapy process. Practice and coaching are integral to changing habits, so support groups and one-to-one visits focused on counseling can produce faster outcomes.

This process of reframing thoughts can be more difficult with patients who only want to believe that there is a physical cause of their symptoms, or who have become rigid in their thoughts and behaviors. It helps to have frequent visits, and to tell patients that the symptom has multiple causes, which require multiple treatments that need to be slowly addressed over time. This message is important for patients who are not used to receiving continuous care for their illnesses.

Medication may be needed for underlying mental health conditions (*see* Chapter 7). Chun-Hua had become significantly incapacitated by anxiety. She was unable to concentrate on her studies, or even on her thoughts. Her doctor prescribed a 6-month trial of medication to reduce her anxiety and improve her concentration so that she could benefit from the cognitive therapy process.

UNIVERSAL COMPONENTS OF HEALTHCARE SYSTEMS

The underlying principles of the Western medical model may be incompatible with healthcare systems in developing countries.[11] These principles may be more implicit than explicit, and include the beliefs that:

1 symptoms are biomedical until proven otherwise

2 the Western medical model is the gold standard to which all other health systems should refer

3 healing is the cure of biomedical symptoms.

The medical model tends to "medicalize" syndromes and illnesses that are usually taken care of by the popular and folk sectors of a developing country's medical system. This tendency is not always in the best interests of our patients. Practitioners can better understand their patients' decisions about their health by finding out who they have gone to for previous treatment for their conditions. The universal treatment components of any country's healthcare system include the professional, folk, and popular sectors.[11]

"Professional" practitioners undergo formal training above and beyond college. They belong to professional organizations that educate, advocate for, and support their members. In Vietnam, the professionals include physicians trained in traditional medicine, the Western medical model, or a combination of both traditional and Western medicine. Other primary healthcare practitioners include assistant physicians, nurses, midwives, and pharmacists. Since 2006, schools of social work have begun to train Bachelor-degree-level students who will be ready to work in the communal health centers. New Master's programs are in the process of development in several urban areas of Vietnam where previously they did not exist. This is the case in many low-income countries.

"Folk" practitioners include non-secular practitioners such as shamans and priests, and secular practitioners such as snake healers, geomancers, bone setters, fortune tellers, herbalists, and palm readers.

The "popular sector" begins with the patient's family. Their knowledge, secrets, and treatments are passed down through generations, and then branch out to friends and acquaintances who share their own family secrets when the patient's family remedies do not work. Folk and popular treatments involve little expense, are readily available in most parts of the developing world, and tend to be consistent with patients' beliefs and values. Over the past 30 years, the Vietnamese government has strongly discouraged people from going to folk healers for health decisions and care. Yet families continue to consult folk healers to choose wedding dates, or names for their children.

In many developing countries, patients rely heavily on the folk and popular sectors, and may never see a Western-trained healthcare practitioner during their lifetime. In China, patients are likely to have seen five practitioners from the popular and folk sectors before they ever consult a medical doctor. In most developing countries, continuity of care is virtually non-existent.[11] In Vietnam, if symptoms are not resolved within one or two visits, patients seek care from other medical practitioners at the district or provincial level, with minimal communication between the healthcare practitioners at the various levels of care.

The type of symptom or complaint influences the patient's decision about where to go first. A patient is likely to seek care from a medical practitioner if symptoms are ongoing and are perceived to have a physical cause. However, they will usually go to folk or popular practitioners if symptoms are perceived to have a psychosocial or spiritual cause.

Cultural beliefs can prevent patients from obtaining or adhering to effective treatment. Therefore healthcare practitioners should try to assess patients' beliefs from the very beginning in order to discover influences that may have a negative impact on care, treatment, and follow-up.

ELICITING EXPLANATORY MODELS

A strategic way to understand patients' cultural beliefs is to explore their *explanatory model* – that is, the set of ideas that they have about their illness.[12] If the explanatory models of the patient, the family, and the healthcare practitioner are in agreement, there is a good chance that the patient will follow through with the recommended treatment. If the explanatory models are not in agreement, the patient will be less likely to follow through with the treatment recommendations. In cultures where there is no continuity of care, and physicians are treated with unquestioning deference, practitioners will not know whether the patient agrees or disagrees with their recommendations. The patient will not be open and honest about their different explanatory model, for fear of offending their practitioner.

Therefore it is very important for healthcare practitioners to make the implicit disagreements explicit. Practitioners need to create a safe environment in which different viewpoints can be discussed, so that common ground can be found and healing can begin to take place.

Physicians can incorporate the following questions at extended office visits or over the course of several visits:

1 What are your ideas about the illness (e.g. the cause, contributing factors, why it is occurring now)?
2 What are your feelings about and reactions to having this illness?
3 What are the effects of the illness on your life?
4 What are your expectations of today's visit, the course of the illness, or treatment?

Nurses, social workers, or community workers may have more time to spend with patients, and can ask the following additional questions in order to obtain more detailed information:

1 Do you have a specific name for your problem?
2 What are you thoughts about why it began when it did?
3 What are your beliefs about its severity and duration?
4 What troubles you most about your sickness?
5 What treatments have you already tried and what have been the effects of these treatments?
6 What are your hopes for this treatment?[11]

FINDING COMMON GROUND WITH PATIENTS

Physicians and other healthcare practitioners go into medicine because they want to be healers and they want to be able to transform patients' lives for the better. Unfortunately, many medical systems and training programs do not support this role. Practitioners often find themselves in the role of highly trained technicians, doing nothing more than treating presenting symptoms. This does not have to be the case. Lang and colleagues have outlined strategies that promote finding common ground between patient and practitioner when they explicitly or implicitly disagree about treatment.[13] These same strategies can be used when the differences are more subtle, or when the patient is not so willing to talk about the differences. The strategies listed below assume that the practitioner has already uncovered the patient's explanatory model and has identified a potential conflict between the patient's and the practitioner's perspectives.

1 **Acknowledge, validate, and explore the patient's explanatory model** and how it differs from your own.
2 **Explore the patient's motivation** to do what is necessary to get better, using the patient's values to help to motivate them. In Marguerite's case, she had two small children at home. Her practitioner told her that her children needed her to get better, and that doing everything she could to take control of her symptoms would really help her children.
3 **Options:**
  — **Collaborate with the patient's explanatory model,** brainstorming options that include the perspective and interests of both yourself and the patient. If there is sufficient time, identify the benefits and drawbacks of continuing behaviors, along with incentives and obstacles to changing behaviors (*see* Chapter 4).
  — **Compromise:** If the patient gives in on one thing, you give in on something else, so that you may come closer to agreement.
  — **Set criteria** to decide between two or more options. For example, if the patient wants medication that you think is inappropriate, what criteria would indicate that the use of that medication is indeed appropriate?
4 **Assess the patient's willingness and ability** to carry out the plan (*see* Chapter 4).
5 **Clarify the mutual responsibilities** of yourself and your patient.[13]

Many factors influence the practitioner's ability to explore the patient's perspectives and explanatory models of their illnesses. If a healthcare system values only the number of patients who are seen by practitioners, there is little incentive to explore patients' explanatory models and underlying psychological diagnoses. There would then be less likelihood that treatable psychological conditions or cognitive distortions would be uncovered, or that social contributors to the patients' illnesses would be dealt with effectively. In such systems, patients with a high level of psychosocial issues and physical complaints will not be treated adequately, and will go from one practitioner to another, never improving, increasing health costs, and with an increased likelihood of becoming disabled by inappropriate care and poor choices.

GUIDING PRINCIPLES

We recognize that many practitioners might initially feel uncomfortable discussing explanatory models and family stresses with patients. The following guiding principles may provide both patients and practitioners with a sense of safety:

1   **Integrate biomedical and psychosocial questions** from the very beginning, no matter what the concern.

2   **Listen**, and don't argue, no matter how different the patient's perspective is from yours. If you react too quickly to patients' different views and opinions, they may become defensive, they may feel that they are not being listened to, and they may not pay attention to your recommendations.

3   **Work towards establishing a collaborative partnership** with the patient. This may be more difficult in some cultures and with some patients. In Vietnam, for example, many patients have spent most of their lives under a communist government and have also been heavily influenced by Confucianism. Both of these thought systems are very proscriptive about who makes decisions. Patients are taught to honor physicians, so they expect to be told what to do, and would consider it very inappropriate to openly disagree with the doctor. Even in cultures with less proscriptive traditions, there will always be some patients who want you to tell them what to do.

4   **Explore the patient's current status and life history** in order to understand their stressors and response patterns. This can be done over the course of multiple visits.

5   **Build bridges** between the patient's explanatory models and yours in order to create effective treatment plans. This involves finding common ground between your perspective and that of your patient.

6   **Manage time and the conversation in order to prioritize** what is discussed during each visit. Bring the patient back for other visits. A continuity-of-care relationship that follows the patient's illness, stories, and progress over time is essential in primary care.

CONCLUSION

This chapter has described how healthcare practitioners can work with patients whose physical health is compromised by stress. It provides clear strategies and guidelines for working with such patients. Necessary conditions are described to blend practitioners' and patients' explanatory models, increasing the likelihood that agreement on treatment and care will be reached. By honoring their patients' beliefs, practitioners increase the likelihood that they will become true healers of their patients.

KEY RESOURCES

- **Benson–Henry Institute for Mind Body Medicine:** provides mind–body resources and courses to reduce stress and also to reduce the effects of stress on the body; www.mbmi.org/home
- **World Federation for Mental Health:** a non-profit global alliance of national

mental health organizations that provides advocacy and education to consumers and medical practitioners. Many of its educational documents have been translated into multiple languages; www.mentalhealthngo. org/users/NGOCommittee3033/docs//World%20Federation%20for%20 Mental%20Health.htm

REFERENCES

1 World Health Organization. *International Classification of Diseases, 10th Revision (ICD-10)*. Geneva: World Health Organization; 1992.

2 American Psychiatric Association. *Diagnostic and Statistical Manual of Mental Disorders, Fourth Edition, Text Revision (DSM-IV-TR)*. Washington, DC: American Psychiatric Association; 2000.

3 Guarnaccia PJ, Rogler LH. Research on culture-bound syndromes: new directions. *Am J Psychiatry*. 1999; **159**: 1322–7.

4 Schwartz PY. Why is neurasthenia important in Asian cultures? *West J Med*. 2002; **176**: 257–8.

5 Chinese Medical Association. *Chinese Classification of Mental Disorders, 2nd Edition, Revised (CCMD-2-R)*. Nanjing, China: Dong Nan University Press; 1995.

6 Selye H. *The Stress of Life*. Columbus, OH: McGraw-Hill; 1978.

7 Benson H. *The Relaxation Response*. New York: Harper Collins Publishers; 2000.

8 Borysenko J. *Minding the Body, Mending the Mind*. Reading, MA: Addison-Wesley Publishing Co.; 1987.

9 World Health Organization. *Mental Disorders in Primary Care*; http://whqlibdoc.who. int/HQ/1998/WHO_MSA_MNHIEAC_98.1.pdf (accessed 8 January 2009).

10 Hodge DR, Nadir A. Culturally competent practice with Muslims: modifying cognitive therapy with Islamic tenets. *Soc Work*. 2008; **53**: 31–41.

11 Kleinman A. *Patients and Healers in the Context of Culture: an exploration of the borderland between anthropology, medicine, and psychiatry*. Berkeley, CA: University of California Press; 1980.

12 Kleinman A. *The Illness Narratives: suffering, healing and the human condition*. New York: Basic Books; 1988.

13 Lang F, Floyd M, Bein K, *et al. Reaching Common Ground: core communication skills of a patient-centered clinical interview*. Johnson City, TN: Department of Family Medicine, East Tennessee State University; 2001.

CHAPTER 4

Behavioral change

Julie M Schirmer, Kimberly Green and Nguyen Vu Quoc Huy

> ### CASE SCENARIO
>
> Selan is a 19-year-old Ethiopian mother who brings her first-born, 3-month-old son to the health clinic because of diarrhea that has lasted over a week. The mother is concerned because he seems to be losing weight. He was born at home with a deformed right leg. They had named him Mengesha, which means "kingdom." Selan's family is struggling, as the grandparents and other relatives believe that the deformity is due to an evil spell that had been cast on Mengesha.

INTRODUCTION

This chapter describes strategies and brief interventions that healthcare practitioners can use to promote health and to reduce risk and harm. These simple tools include questions about the importance of the problem to the patient and their commitment to change, a decision analysis and other motivational interviewing strategies. The chapter describes how these models apply to Selan and Mengesha's family and to others whose health would dramatically improve if they made healthier choices.

Unhealthy beliefs, behaviors, and choices of people contribute to more than 50% of conditions that are treated in primary care sites.[1] Tobacco use, alcohol and other drug misuse, and unsafe sexual practices directly affect the health and safety of patients and their families, and might reasonably be considered contributing factors to Mengesha's illness. Primary healthcare practitioners have a leading role to play in preventing and treating disease and helping patients to make the necessary lifestyle changes to improve their health and the health of their family.

Only about one-third of patients change unhealthy behaviors after learning that their behaviors will harm them.[2] Healthcare practitioners must use relationship-building skills and intervention models to empower the other two-thirds to make the changes that are needed to improve their health.

We recognize that many factors contribute to poor health and unhealthy choices and are not under an individual's control (e.g. war, poverty, environmental influences, and lack of community resources such as education and healthcare services). Exposure of an individual to abuse and other adverse childhood experiences sets them up for increased risky behaviors, high rates of mental and chronic health disorders, and a tendency to believe that outside influences are in control of their health. These factors are extremely important, and they require systemic changes that can best be addressed through public health and community health measures (*see* community-oriented primary care principles in Chapter 8).

SIMPLE TOOLS FOR COMPLEX SITUATIONS

Healthcare practitioners need to have the skills to successfully address complex situations. Such complex situations are common among people from countries where poverty is high and where there is lack of support to help care for dependent family members. Physical or mental disabilities in families can reduce their ability to function. Patients with such disabilities and their families learn to change to a more realistic and functional way of interacting with the world around them. In Mengesha's case, the illness is difficult to treat, especially since the mother may not be able to read well enough to follow feeding instructions precisely. While the healthcare practitioner was inquiring about the baby's nutrition and immediate health history, she discovered that the mother was concerned that someone was poisoning her son.

> At birth, Selan's relatives had encouraged her to poison her baby or abandon him in the forest. This was common practice in her village when children were born with physical deformities. Selan and her husband did not believe in the evil spell theory of Mengesha's deformity, and had decided to do everything possible to give Mengesha a chance to survive. The elders in the village were trying to persuade them to send Mengesha to an orphanage in a town 100 kilometers away.[3]

The healthcare practitioner was from a nearby village and was aware of similar situations. Through the history, the practitioner discovered that Selan was using infant formula but was not sterilizing her bottles properly. Selan was very tearful during the visit. The practitioner was concerned about Selan's possible depression and how it could affect her outlook and her ability to care for herself and her infant son (*see* Chapter 7). This was a rural health center, where the practitioner had plenty of time to devote to this mother and child. If it had been a busy urban hospital clinic, where the average time spent with patients is 3 to 5 minutes, she would not have had as much opportunity to address these issues.

Since she did have the time, this practitioner *framed* the discussion with Selan to promote behavior change and empower this new mother, who was very protective of Mengesha and wanted to show that she was able to care for him.[4] The FRAMES model provides healthcare practitioners with a way to be therapeutic in a time-efficient manner, without taking on an overwhelming amount of detail.

Practitioners can "open the window" that sheds light on the psychosocial contributors to a patient's illness, and can then "close the window" in a therapeutic manner that is helpful to patients.

We recognize that the FRAMES model and several other tools in this book are based on words or phrases that make sense in English, but which may not make sense when translated into other languages. We hope that those who work in the non-English-speaking parts of the world will be able to modify the acronym to make sense in their own language, but in a way that maintains the integrity of the model. The FRAMES model[5] consists of the following elements:

➤ Feedback
➤ Responsibility of patient
➤ Advice
➤ Menu of options
➤ Empathy
➤ Self-efficacy.

F stands for personalized *feedback* from the patient's perspective. In this case, the feedback is what Selan and her family believed was the cause of the illness, and her expectations about how it should be treated. Errors in thinking can be identified and addressed during the discussion.

R stands for the patient's *responsibility* for making decisions about the baby's care.

A stands for the *advice* given by the practitioner. In this case, it is the advice that the practitioner gave Selan about correct sterilizing techniques, about which antibiotics to use, and about what to do if her baby's condition worsened. She then used pictures to show Selan how to administer the medicine, and finished by asking her to tell her how she would follow through with instructions at home.

M stands for a *menu* of options.

> The practitioner was concerned about this new mother and baby. She gave Selan enough antibiotics for three days, with instructions to then bring Mengesha to the clinic to receive more medication. The practitioner also offered to make a home visit, which would provide an opportunity to meet with Selan and the family elders to address current issues and offer them some hope about the infant's healthy development. She shared information about health clinics and other supports for Mengesha that would eventually provide a leg prosthesis and vocational training in a nearby city.

E stands for *empathy* ("I know this is really difficult, and you are very concerned").

Finally, S stands for *self-efficacy* – in this case, the patient's confidence in making the changes necessary to improve the health both of her baby and of herself ("You are such a good mother. You brought him to the clinic before he could get any worse").

This mother had recived no healthcare during her pregnancy, nor had she had the help of any practitioner during the birth. This practitioner would use motivational interviewing skills to persuade her to come to the clinic for vitamins and shots for her baby, and for advice on the use of folic acid and vitamins during her next pregnancy, to reduce the likelihood of birth abnormalities and allow her to produce the healthiest infant possible.

This scenario demonstrates how complex the obstacles can be when changing health behaviors and practices. The grandparents' beliefs and community practices were working against this mother in even bringing her child to receive care at the clinic. It was critically important for the healthcare practitioner not only to help this infant and mother, but also to help the family and community elders to recognize the benefits of prenatal care, medically attended deliveries, and healthcare of infants and children even when they are not ill.

Many factors can complicate the change process, such as addictions, mental health issues, and limited individual autonomy, especially among people with limited education, scarce employment opportunities, or dependency (self-imposed or otherwise). Where people are weakened due to war, extreme poverty, forced dependence on family, or unhealthy employment options (e.g. sex workers or drug dealers), referrals to community empowerment programs help to provide support and other options once the unhealthy habits have been changed. Available options may include community clubs to support healthy habits, advocacy opportunities to educate and influence others, and retraining/employment opportunities.

HEALTH PROMOTION AND RISK REDUCTION COUNSELING

A large part of primary care practice in the developed world is focused on health promotion and risk reduction activities. Health promotion activities enable people to take control of their own health, and include counseling about diet for people with diabetes, exercise for obese or depressed patients, and social activities for those who are isolated due to bereavement or depression. Risk reduction activities attempt to bring some measure of self-control over disease processes to moderate- or high-risk patients.

Risk reduction activities include assessing and addressing high-risk behaviors such as the use of cigarettes, alcohol, or drugs. Brief interventions by primary care physicians, lasting less than 5 minutes, have been shown to be effective in helping patients to quit smoking.[6] The Five A's model for smoking cessation counseling is an easy-to-remember mnemonic that has had demonstrated success in primary care (*see* Table 4.1). For those who are unwilling to quit, the Five R's model can help to increase motivation (*see* Table 4.2). The Five A's and the Five R's models can be easily applied to other types of behavioral changes that patients need to make to improve their health.

TABLE 4.1 The 5 A's model for smoking cessation

Ask about tobacco use at every visit.

Advise every smoker to quit.

Advice should be clear, strong, and personalized.

Assess the patient's willingness to quit.

Scale the patient's motivation to quit. Begin the decision analysis process (risks and benefits of quitting and not quitting).

Assist the patient in their attempts to quit.

Establish a quit plan and date.

Change the patient's environment to decrease triggers and obtain access to support.

Provide information about addiction, the importance of abstinence, and withdrawal symptoms.

Provide pharmacotherapy, if available.

Include self-help materials (*see* Key Resources at end of chapter).

Arrange for follow-up, preferably 1 week after quitting, 1 month thereafter, and then as needed.

Congratulate the patient.

Discuss relapse potential (to prevent, normalize, and problem-solve).

Adapted from Fiore MC, Carlos RJC, Baker TR, *et al. Strategies A1–A5*. Rockville, MD: Public Health Service, US Department of Health and Human Services, 2008. Available from the National Library of Medicine (www.ncbi.nlm.nih.gov/books/bv.fcgi?rid=hstat2.chapter.28163) and from the Office of the Surgeon General (www.surgeongeneral.gov/tobacco/treating_tobacco_use08.pdf)

TABLE 4.2 The Five R's model for enhancing patient motivation

The Five R's	Clinical strategies
Relevance	Explore why quitting is personally relevant to the patient (e.g. impacting an existing disease process, the family or social situation, or other health concerns).
	Inquire about previous quit attempts to inform current treatment.
Risk	Ask the patient to identify potential negative consequences of smoking.
Rewards	Ask the patient about potential benefits of quitting smoking.
	Point out rewards. For example:
	• improves health
	• reduces effect of "second-hand smoke" on family
	• sets a good example for children
	• means more money is available for other things
	• makes food taste better
	• improves sense of smell.
Roadblocks	Ask the patient to identify barriers to quitting, and problem-solve about them.
Repetition	Repeat parts of intervention at every visit.

Adapted from Fiore MC, Carlos RJC, Baker TR, *et al. Strategies B1 and B2*. Rockville, MD: Public Health Service, US Department of Health and Human Services, 2008. Available from the National Library of Medicine (www.ncbi.nlm.nih.gov/books/bv.fcgi?rid=hstat2.chapter.28163) and from the Office of the Surgeon General (www.surgeongeneral.gov/tobacco/treating_tobacco_use08.pdf)

MOTIVATIONAL INTERVIEWING AND THE STAGES OF CHANGE

Marjani is a 27-year-old woman who is visited by the home-based care team linked to a local district hospital in Kenya. She has severe pelvic pain and is in need of care. From her history and exam the patient appears to be an injecting drug user who, the home-based care team suspects, has a sexually transmitted infection that appears to be the cause of the pain. She has been self-treating with an antibiotic that she bought at the local store and that has not been effective. Ever since her husband died from HIV two years ago, Marjani has been employed as a sex worker to support her drug habit and her two small children. Her family refuses to acknowledge her or to provide any kind of support. She and her children live in a slum dwelling with other sex workers. She does not have enough money to send her oldest child to school. The home-based care team cannot make a diagnosis and therefore needs to refer Marjani to the district hospital for a full examination and treatment. She is fearful that the medical practitioner will inform the authorities, but she desperately needs help to relieve her pain, which is affecting her functioning and livelihood. She is also worried that she cannot afford to pay for care at the local hospital.

Motivational interviewing is a way of discussing change that can help Marjani. It reduces patient resistance, enhances intrinsic motivation to change, and promotes self-efficacy. The aim is to inspire patients to make the changes that are necessary in order to improve their health. This form of counseling has proved successful in improving treatment of substance abuse, adherence to medication and diet, and prevention of infectious and chronic disease.[7] In developing countries, motivational interviewing has proved effective in addressing intravenous drug use, high-risk sexual behaviors, and the use of safe water systems.[8] In countries where there are high death rates from traffic accidents, the method can be used to increase the use of seatbelts and motorcycle helmets.

Motivational interviewing views change as a continuum of stages that patients go through in order to improve their health.[9] The healthcare practitioner uses directed interventions or strategies, depending on the patient's stage of change. As the patient progresses through the stages, the practitioner response evolves from initially addressing gaps in knowledge, to addressing attitudes and motivation to change, to finally suggesting behavioral change options (*see* Table 4.3). Employing any of these strategies too early or at the wrong time can lead to patient resistance.

Patients begin at the *precontemplation* stage, where they are unaware of or deny the severity of the contribution of their behaviors to their health issues. At this stage, they are not considering giving up the habit or changing unhealthy behaviors. The *contemplation* stage occurs when the patient begins to consider making the necessary changes. The *preparation* stage occurs when they have the vision to change, but do not yet possess the skills necessary to change. Minor attempts at behavioral change occur, but they are not long-lasting. The *action* stage occurs when the patient has the vision, motivation, skills, and plan to change their behavior. This model recognizes relapse when there is a return to the problem behavior, after a sustained resolution. By identifying an explicit stage for relapse, this model recognizes relapse as a normal part of the process. Habits that have been practiced over a lifetime are difficult to change. After initial attempts, most patients tend to revert to unhealthy behaviors, otherwise known as "relapse." If their habits are deeply entrenched, it may take five to seven attempts to change before they reach the *maintenance* stage. This stage describes patients who have succeeded in giving up the unhealthy behaviors and are determined to maintain their success.

There are multiple barriers to the movement of a patient from one stage to another. In Marjani's case, the factors that limit her ability to change her sexual practices include addiction, a possible mental health problem such as depression, lack of other opportunities to provide for her family, and little autonomy working in the commercial sex world. Unfortunately, such situations are not uncommon where economic resources are scarce and people may worry about where the next meal is coming from. As we shall see later in this chapter, family and community beliefs can undermine healthy behaviors. When barriers to change are complicated and risks are high, it is important for community providers and volunteer networks to provide support to patients and to be familiar with the stages of change model.

APPLICATION

Table 4.3 describes specific skills that practitioners can use to help patients to progress through the five stages of the motivational interviewing model. The table highlights the 5 A's model of addressing change. Guiding principles include the following:
1 using empathy
2 developing a discrepancy between beliefs that contribute to unhealthy choices and the evidence that challenges such beliefs
3 rolling with patient resistance to change
4 supporting self-efficacy (people's belief that they can make the changes necessary to improve their health)
5 enabling an environment for change by using brief counseling skills at each encounter.

TABLE 4.3 Patients' readiness to change and treatment strategies

Stage	General description	Goal	Strategy
Precontemplation	Denies or is unaware of the problem; is resistant, defensive, or unmotivated	Increase awareness of benefits; increase knowledge; create ambivalence	**Ask** what the patient knows about the effects on their health; gently point out the risks and problems; express concern; provide educational materials

(continued)

Stage	General description	Goal	Strategy
Contemplation	Is ambivalent; aware of reasons, but perceives many barriers to change; costs outweigh benefits	Motivate, reduce barriers, and enhance self-efficacy	**Advise:** help to identify the pros and cons of change; problem-solve barriers; suggest "mini-trials" of new behavior
Preparation	Intends to take action; begins to form commitment to specific goal, methods and timetable	Discuss, encourage and support the patient in making changes; identify critical factors for success	**Assist:** Assess patient's confidence and problem-solve barriers; identify useful social supports; encourage start date; set gradual, realistic goals
Action	Has recently made changes; may not yet have met goals; has not sustained change; is vulnerable to abandoning effort impulsively	Help patient to continue to make changes; provide feedback and support	**Arrange:** remind patient of the benefits of change; identify high-risk situations and coping strategies; reinforce changes to date
Maintenance	Has sustained change for more than 6 weeks; works towards preventing relapse; high confidence in sustaining goal behavior	Help to sustain health risk reduction	**Ask** about feelings and how expectations have been met; show support and admiration; support lifestyle that reduces risk of relapse
Relapse	Consistent return to problem behavior after resolution	Normalize relapse as a learning opportunity and part of the long-standing process of change	**Ask** about the specifics of change and relapse; praise willingness to change; assist in finding other coping strategies

Adapted from deGruy FV, Perry Dickinson W, Staton EW. *20 Common Problems in Behavioral Health.* New York: McGraw-Hill; 2001.

The following case scenario demonstrates how these techniques helped one patient to quit smoking:

Ibrahim is a 50-year-old man who comes to the primary care clinic for a worsening chronic cough, which keeps him awake at night and contributes to his fatigue. He continues to smoke, despite this cough, chronic sinusitis, shortness of breath, fatigue, and insomnia. He owns a taxi company, but his ill health is making it very difficult for him to work. Ibrahim comes to the clinic with his wife, Afsah, who is very worried about him.

After exam and work-up, the practitioner told Ibrahim that he had a lung condition (chronic obstructive pulmonary disease) that was caused or made worse by his smoking. Ibrahim appeared upset and said that his parents and grandparents were all smokers and lived long and healthy lives. He stated that his father had recently died from quitting smoking, because he had had a stroke one month after quitting smoking, and died shortly thereafter. The practitioner acknowledged Ibrahim's grief and commented on how his father's situation could affect his outlook on quitting (empathy). The practitioner briefly pointed out that Ibrahim's father's 40-year smoking history had certainly damaged his cardiovascular system and placed him at greater risk of having a stroke. The practitioner used Ibrahim's lab and X-ray results as evidence that his continued smoking was having a harmful effect on his body (developing discrepancy). He said that he cared about Ibrahim and was concerned that continued smoking would only make his symptoms worse (empathy). He also acknowledged that most of his patients thought that quitting smoking was the most difficult thing they had ever had to do (rolling with resistance).

After providing Ibrahim with medication to help to minimize his symptoms, the practitioner said, "When you are ready to quit, there is help available and we can be part of that help." Ibrahim was clearly in the *precontemplation* stage. During the office interview, he progressed from arriving in an angry and defensive mood to leaving a little more thoughtful and informed about the effects of his smoking.

Several months later, Ibrahim returned with similar symptoms and a request for more medication. He showed interest in stopping smoking, but was afraid that he could not follow through. He had made several meager attempts to do so, but they were fairly impulsive and unsuccessful. Ibrahim was moving towards the *contemplation* stage. After treating his symptoms, the doctor arranged for the nurse to meet with him.

The nurse explored the reasons why Ibrahim was considering quitting. What were the pros and cons of quitting? What troubled him the most about continuing to smoke or about quitting? Ibrahim was worried about being too sick to provide for his family, and was fearful that he would not be able to watch his grandchildren grow up. He agreed to make a list, over the next couple of weeks, of the pros and cons of continuing smoking and of quitting, and he returned to see the nurse (*see* Table 4.4). This formal "decision analysis" helped Ibrahim to make his thinking process and feelings more explicit, and incorporated the opinions of medical experts and concerned family and friends into his worldview. It played a part in tipping the balance from the contemplative to the preparation stage.

The decision analysis unearthed many of Ibrahim's values with regard to his family and his ability to provide for them. Everyone shows discrepancies in their values between what they say and what they do. The nurse helped Ibrahim to start to make a list of what he valued, such as quitting smoking and taking care of his parents, wife, and children. He completed the list at home and brought it back to show the nurse at a later visit, when they reviewed the discrepancy between what he said he valued and what he actually did in relation to those values. Deep change requires a guiding compass. Uncovering what is most important to a person, or what they value, can help motivate a patient towards improved health behaviors.

TABLE 4.4 Decision analysis*

Staying the same (not changing behavior)	Reasons for changing behavior
What are the benefits of your unhealthy habit?	What are your concerns about your unhealthy habit?
What are your concerns about changing your unhealthy habit?	What are the benefits of changing your unhealthy habit?

Adapted from Botelho R. *Motivational Practice: promoting healthy habits and self-care of chronic diseases.* New York: MHH Publications; 2004.

*To watch how to use a decision balance, go to www.motivatehealthyhabits.com/smoking-old/task1. php3?slidenum=01

Over the course of Ibrahim's visits, the nurse asked him to assess how important smoking was for him, using a scale of 1 to 10 (where 10 was the most important problem he had ever experienced, and 1 was the least important). Using similar scales, she then asked him "How committed are you to stopping smoking?" and "How confident are you about following through with your commitment to stop?" If his confidence was less than 7 (on a scale of 1 to 10 where 10 was most confident), they would either alter his goal (cut down or quit), or brainstorm about the obstacles that could get in his way. These questions were instrumental in identifying where Ibrahim was in relation to the stages. The nurse helped him to identify potential barriers, dangerous triggers and situations to avoid, effective coping strategies, and a reasonable time frame for him to cut down and then quit altogether. After a number of visits, Ibrahim eventually asked if ongoing assistance was available to help him to quit smoking. He had made several previous attempts, but on each occasion could only stop for two or three days.

If there was an underlying anxiety disorder, Ibrahim's condition might worsen if he even just thought about quitting smoking. If he was receiving care at a hospital clinic, a psychiatrist, social worker, or psychologist might meet with him to assess and treat any underlying mental health conditions.

This healthcare team was able to stay in contact with Ibrahim because he continued to have health crises related to his smoking. They supported him through his relapses (which they normalized), helped to identify barriers, found solutions to problems, and provided support and encouragement. They asked him for details about his relapses to help him to become more conscious of obstacles and how to plan ways around them. During the maintenance stage, they identified new activities that would take him away from high-risk smoking situations (bars and long lunches with his co-workers) and into healthy, generative activities, such as spending more time riding his bike and weeding the family garden.

Follow-up is extremely important. Regardless of why the patient is seeking care, healthcare practitioners can continue to inquire about healthy behavioral changes to promote the patient's advancement through the stages of change, assist with relapses, and promote a sense of pride once the change has taken place to protect the patient's health and that of their families.

CONCLUSION

Behavioral change theories and models are essential for helping healthcare practitioners and community providers to address patients' risky behaviors. Primary care physicians can screen and incorporate brief counseling techniques at each visit. Nurses, social workers, psychologists, and psychiatrists may have more time to focus on unhealthy behaviors, and are likely to have both the skills and the time for more intensive counseling. Paraprofessionals working in the community can use behavioral change interventions to support patients in settings that are closer to home or even in the home. Each level of care can enhance what the others are doing to improve the overall health of their communities.

KEY RESOURCES

- **Motivational Interviewing:** includes information about the approach, links, training resources, reprints, and recent research (William R Miller, PhD and Stephen Rollnick, PhD); www.motivationalinterview.org
- **Motivate Healthy Habits: empowering individuals, families and communities:** a website with resources for health practitioners, including complimentary chapters of key books, articles, presentations, and support materials for practitioners on smoking cessation, excessive alcohol use, and self-care of diabetes (Rick Botelho, MD); www.motivatehealthyhabits.com/index.html
- **Family Health International** is an organization dedicated to improving the health and welfare of individuals and families in resource-poor parts of the world. Guidelines, training resources, and toolkits are available for healthcare workers, people living with progressive chronic diseases such as HIV, and people who engage in sex work, drug use, and unprotected sex; www.fhi.org
- **The Alcohol Clinical Training (ACT) Project:** provides information on the latest research, curriculum, and pragmatic clinical skills for screening and conducting brief interventions for alcohol problems; www.bu.edu/act/mdalcoholtraining/index/html
- **The CHANGE Project:** provides programmatic and educational resources for behavioral change innovation, tools, and strategies focusing on health and nutrition programs; www.changeproject.org/index.html

REFERENCES

1 World Health Organization. *The World Health Report 2002. Reducing risks, promoting healthy life*; www.who.int/whr/2002/en/ (accessed 15 January 2008).
2 Bazata DD, Robinson JG, Fox KM, *et al.* Affecting behavioral change in individuals with diabetes. *Diabetes Educ.* 2008; **34:** 1025–36.
3 Lax L, Stern N. *Emmanuel's Gift.* USA, 2005, 80 minutes.
4 Velasquez MM. *You do WHAT research in a Family Medicine Department? Transtheoretical model of change.* Annual Conference of the Society of Teachers of Family Medicine, 12–16 May 2004, Toronto, ON.
5 Miller WR, Rollnick S. *Motivational Interviewing: preparing people to change addictive behavior.* New York: Guilford Press; 1991 (reprinted with permission of Guilford Press).
6 Fiore MC, Roberto C, Jaén C, *et al. Treating Tobacco Use and Dependence: clinical practice guidelines. 2008 update.* Rockville, MD: Agency for Healthcare Research and Quality, US Department of Health and Human Resources; 2008; www.ahrq.gov/clinic/tobacco/tobaqrg.htm (accessed 18 May 2009).
7 Botelho R. *Motivational Interviewing: stepping stones to lasting change.* New York: MHH Publications; 2004.
8 Thevos A, Kaona F, Siajunza M, *et al.* Adoption of safe water behaviors in Zambia: comparing educational and motivational approaches. *Educ Health.* 2000; **13:** 366–76.
9 Prochaska JO, Velicer WF. The transtheoretical model of health behavior change. *Am J Health Promot.* 1997; **12:** 38–48.

CHAPTER 5

Family systems in behavioral health*

Alan Lorenz, Julie M Schirmer, Nguyen Thi Kim Chuc and Nguyen Van Hung

CASE SCENARIO

Pham Thi Minh is a 53-year-old Vietnamese woman who reluctantly presents to her healthcare practitioner with headaches and fatigue. She has been referred by her neighbor and good friend who is concerned about her increasing symptoms. Her headaches have been getting worse over the past 6 months and are associated with irritability and sensitivity to light. The headaches are relieved by rest in a dark room. The second concern, fatigue, has been slowly progressing over a similar span of time and is generalized and non-specific. After obtaining a brief history of her present illness, her healthcare practitioner seeks "background information" using a genogram as a template for the family and personal history.

(The Vietnamese order for naming is used here, with family names listed first and given names listed second.)

INTRODUCTION

At our core, we are relational beings, and our most important relationships are with our family. Relationships with our parents and siblings form the basis of our future relationships. Eventually, friends, and then colleagues, further embellish our lives. Often our relationships with our spouse or partner, and then potentially with our children and even our grandchildren, constitute much of the fabric of our lives. Since most of us get our ideas about how families function from our own families, our families of origin serve as the standard by which we measure other families. Healthcare practitioners can be trained to develop more complex ideas about family. However, all of our assumptions and emotions come with us

---

* A considerable amount of conceptual material for this chapter appears in another publication of one of the co-authors: McDaniel S, Campbell T, Hepworth J, Lorenz A. *Family-Oriented Primary Care.* 2nd ed. New York: Springer; 2005.

when we meet families professionally, requiring us to monitor our own personal and cultural biases as we consider each family and their response to an illness or new challenge.

Attention to family context is a critical component to understanding every patient's health status. Although the structure and functioning of a family can contribute to overall health and well-being, family problems can also contribute to a wide array of physical and mental disorders. Family characteristics interact with genetic predispositions to affect psychosocial functioning, response to stress, and poor health behaviors. For some acute, self-limited illnesses, a primarily biomedical intervention may be sufficient treatment for a symptom. However, for many medical problems, understanding the web of relationships – the relational context – among family and friends is integral to successful and comprehensive treatment.

With the right skills, healthcare practitioners can assess the structure, development, and functioning of a family easily and quickly. The structure of a family can be illustrated graphically with a genogram diagram (described below) that provides extensive information at a glance. Family development relates to the family members' ages and developmental stages and can be derived from a genogram. Family function is assessed through history and observation of family process. For example, at any visit, a healthcare practitioner can observe whether a parent or partner is comforting to the patient, or whether family members seem to be supportive of one another. Over time and with more complicated medical problems, patients inevitably describe their family functioning as they discuss stresses and coping strategies. Furthermore, as people live longer with more complex problems, families will increasingly be involved with patient care, and healthy family functioning will become even more important.

This chapter begins by describing the basic family systems concepts, which include key family characteristics, structure, process, and the life cycle. Specific questions that healthcare practitioners can ask are embedded in each section. These questions can also be applied to our own families, to uncover our own biases and assumptions about the families that we see. To demonstrate how to integrate family assessment into clinical care, we shall apply them to Minh's family. Later in the chapter, we shall discuss general principles for family interviewing and provide a broad outline for conducting goal-oriented family conferences. We shall use the definition of family as "a group of people related by blood or choice who move together through time."[1] This definition embraces the wider range of intimate family structures that is seen across all cultures.

FAMILY CHARACTERISTICS

Although each family is unique, every family can be understood in terms of a few universal concepts. Table 5.1 depicts key characteristics and questions that a healthcare practitioner can use to explore family stability, family transition, family world view, and the relational context of an illness.

TABLE 5.1 General family characteristics

General family characteristic	Key questions for healthcare practitioners
Family stability: an interpersonal process by which the family strives to maintain emotional balance in the system.	• With all of the changes, what has the family done to maintain balance?
Family transition: an interpersonal process by which the family adapts to developmental growth in members, and to varying expectations and roles in the community.	• How has your family had to adapt to these new developments (e.g. now that your mother-in-law has moved in with you)?
Family worldview: the general view that family members have of themselves as competent or ineffective, cohesive or fragmented. This view can be enhanced when they feel that they have coped with a crisis well, or when a healthcare practitioner recognizes their efforts and affirms their strengths.	• Does your family generally feel that you are able to help one another out in a crisis? • How has it worked when you have had to "fill in" for one another before? • How do family members let one another know when they need help?
Relational context of a symptom: a symptom is part of a larger family and psychosocial context that can influence and be influenced by that symptom.	• How do the patient's symptoms influence everyone else in the family? • Have you noticed if there are things family members do that make the identified patient take more or less responsibility for her medications?

Adapted with kind permission of Springer Science+Business Media from McDaniel SH, Campbell TL, Hepworth J, *et al. Family-Oriented Primary Care*. 2nd ed. New York: Springer-Verlag; 2005. pp. 32–4.

Using these questions, Minh's healthcare practitioner discovered that she is married to Tam, an ex-soldier who is unemployed and has a small pension. The couple have a 15-year-old boy, Linh, who has been doing well in school and has generally been well behaved. Recently, however, he has become more of a challenge to Minh, and has been staying out later than his parents think is appropriate. To support their income, Minh takes care of five preschool-age children in their home. Sometimes Linh teases or bothers the young children. In addition, Minh is the primary caretaker for her husband's mother, Bich, who moved in two years ago. Bich has multiple medical problems that include diabetes and renal failure for which they are considering kidney dialysis (system characteristics). The nephrologist frequently gives instructions that are complicated and time-consuming.

The practitioner discovered that Minh's headaches began at the time when her husband retired from his military position. His job had required him to be away from home a lot. When asked how things had changed since Tam's retirement (family transition), Minh became tearful. Tam was a perfectionist. He constantly criticized Minh about how she cared for their home and day care – tasks that she had managed very well during the years he had been preoccupied by his work (family stability).

The healthcare practitioner discovered that most of the multiple responsibilities of family, day care, and ailing mother-in-law fell on Minh's shoulders. Since his military retirement, Tam had been unsuccessful in finding other employment. He shopped daily for groceries, yet he spent many hours at lunch with his friends (family transition). Minh was exhausted by her many responsibilities. She felt that her requests for help went unanswered (family worldview). She had found that when she went to bed because of her headaches, Linh helped more with the care of her mother-in-law and Tam helped more around the house (relational context of the illness).

The family transitions of Tam's retirement and Bich's increasing disability were affecting the overall functioning and stability of all of the family members.

FAMILY STRUCTURE

Family structure has an impact on patients' health and healthcare behaviors. Table 5.2 illustrates how to assess the structural characteristics of hierarchy, boundaries, family roles, alliances, and coalitions. Cultural norms influence family structure. For example, in many Western cultures there is often considerable geographical separation between family members. Children may go off to college and end up living far away from their parents. Older adults may live in senior living centers or nursing homes. Minh's household, in which three or four generations live together, is fairly typical of many non-Western families. Members of Minh's extended family live within a short walking distance of one another. Her family members see one another every day. They work together and share meals on a regular basis.

In Minh's family, the way in which decisions are made (hierarchy) has shifted since Tam's retirement. Minh had been the primary decision maker during the years that Tam had spent away from home. Now, Tam felt that it was his duty to approve all decisions (role selection). He had been a person of power in the military, yet he was unfamiliar with how things functioned at home. Bich supported Minh in believing that it was the woman's role to run the household (alliance). Tam felt challenged and would lash out at Minh, belittling her in front of their son. Linh was beginning to treat his mother in a similar manner (coalition). The parent–child boundaries were being challenged for the first time.

TABLE 5.2 Family structural characteristics

Family structural characteristic	Key questions for healthcare practitioners
Hierarchy: how power or authority is distributed within the family.	• Who is overtly and covertly in charge of which decisions in the family system? • Is the family's hierarchy clear and appropriate (parents in charge of their children) or reversed (parents controlled by children)?

(*continued*)

Family structural characteristic	Key questions for healthcare practitioners
Boundaries: define the different functional subgroups in the family (e.g. parents, siblings, grandparents).	• What are the subgroups in the family? • Are the boundaries between subgroups (e.g. parents and children) clear and appropriate, or confused and problematic?
Family role selection: the conscious or unconscious assignment of complimentary roles to members of a family.	• What roles do family members play, and how do these roles relate to one another? • Who fills the role of the family's expert on illness and health? • Who is most often the "sick" member of the family?
Alliance: a positive relationship between any two members of a family.	• What are the important alliances in the family?
Coalition: a relationship between at least three people in which two act together secretly against a third person.	• What coalitions exist in the family? • Who is siding against whom?

Adapted with kind permission of Springer Science+Business Media from McDaniel SH, Campbell TL, Hepworth J, *et al. Family-Oriented Primary Care.* 2nd ed. New York: Springer-Verlag; 2005. pp. 35–8.

FAMILY GENOGRAM

In the developed world, every patient expects that basic family, social, past medical, past surgical and relevant personal history information will be obtained at the initial visit and as appropriate at each subsequent visit. The genogram[2–4] is an efficient tool for healthcare practitioners to obtain and document information about family members' names, relationships, and the overall structure of the family. The genogram provides a visual map of connections between family members. When obtaining the genogram, the healthcare practitioner often discovers useful information about the nature and quality of those relationships. A genogram may reveal repetitive dysfunctional emotional patterns, common medical problems, and other important considerations in the process of evaluation and treatment planning.

A typical genogram includes at least three generations of the family, including gender (circle for females, squares for males), names, ages, marital status (horizontal lines), former marriages (horizontal lines with two slashes), children (vertical line below the marital line), significant illnesses, education, occupations, and dates of traumatic events such as deaths. Household members are located within a broken line (*see* Figure 5.1).

Minh's healthcare practitioner began the genogram during the first visit, and continued to shape it during subsequent visits (*see* Figure 5.2).

FAMILY PROCESS

Family process encompasses the types and patterns of interaction between family members. It can affect a person's emotional and physical health and health behaviors, and is assessed through questioning or observation (*see* Table 5.3). These

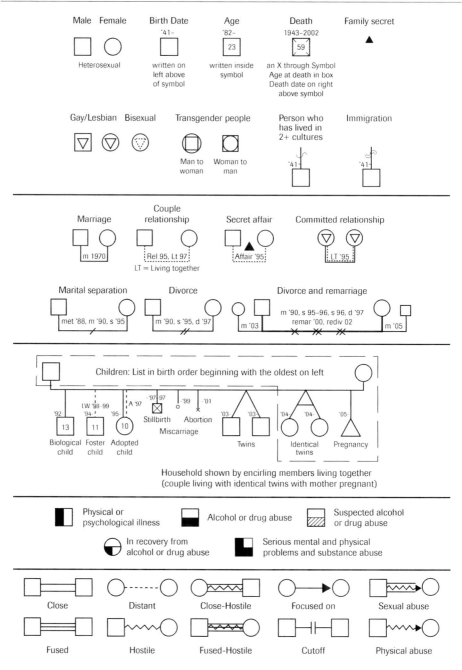

FIGURE 5.1 Common genogram symbols. Reproduced with permission from Monica McGoldrick, LCSW, PhD (hc), Director, Multicultural Family Institute, Highland Park, NJ 08904. *Explaining Genogram Symbols;* www.multiculturalfamily.org/genograms/genogram_symbols.html (accessed 14 March 2009).

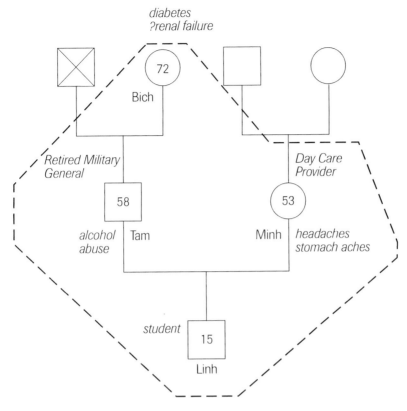

FIGURE 5.2 Minh's family genogram.

interpersonal dynamics often become more pronounced when a family is under stress. A genogram can illustrate family process symbolically. For example, triple lines between members illustrate enmeshment, a line separated by two slashes with a space in between illustrates disengagement, and jagged lines indicate conflict.

TABLE 5.3 Family process characteristics

Family process characteristic	Key questions for healthcare practitioners
Enmeshment: where family members have diminished interpersonal boundaries, limited individual autonomy, and a high degree of emotional reactivity.	• Are family members involved or over-involved with each other? • Do family members "feel each others' feelings"? • Do family members seldom act independently?
Disengagement: where family members are emotionally distant and unresponsive to one another.	• Do family members show little emotional response to each other? Are family members distant or isolated from each other?

(continued)

Family process characteristic	Key questions for healthcare practitioners
Perceived criticism: where family members do not feel valued for their opinions or contributions.	• What happens when you and your family disagree or become stressed? • Does this pattern make the situation better or worse? • If it makes the situation worse, what other behaviors might interrupt the sequence or pattern?

Adapted with kind permission of Springer Science+Business Media from McDaniel SH, Campbell TL, Helworth J, *et al. Family-Oriented Primary Care.* 2nd ed. New York: Springer-Verlag; 2005. pp. 38–9.

> In Minh's case, conflict would best characterize her current relationship with Tam. He was drinking more and was becoming increasingly critical of her. Minh's health-care practitioner was concerned about the impact of this criticism on her health, particularly in view of her increasing medical visits for headaches and fatigue. The practitioner asked Minh what happened when she and Tam disagreed. In tears, Minh relayed that Tam would often come home drunk. More recently he had been punching the walls and throwing things. Minh stated that he was a good man, but that he had become very unhappy since retiring.

FAMILY LIFE CYCLE

The family life cycle (family development) provides a template for quickly assessing the developmental challenges of a patient and their family.[1,5–8] The family life cycle identifies stages of family development that reflect certain cognitive and biological functions. General tasks for families at these stages are described below.

TABLE 5.4 Stages of the family life cycle

Family life cycle stage	Developmental tasks
Leaving home	• Differentiate self in relation to family • Develop intimate peer relationships • Establish oneself in work
Couples and pairing	• Form a committed relationship • Realign relationships with extended family to include partner
Pregnancy and childbirth	• Make room for children in the family • Become parents while remaining partners
Family with young children	• Form a parent team • Negotiate relationships with extended family to include parenting and grandparenting roles

(*continued*)

Family life cycle stage	Developmental tasks
Family with adolescents	• Shift parent–child relationship to permit adolescent to move in and out of system
Adulthood and middle years	• Refocus on marital and career issues • Deal with disabilities and death of grandparents • Deal with own aging and mortality
Graying of the family	• Maintain functioning in the face of physiological decline
Death and grieving	• Deal with loss of partner, siblings, and peers • Prepare for one's own death

Adapted from Carter B. *The Changing Family Life Cycle: a framework for family therapy.* © 1989. Reproduced by permission of Pearson Education, Inc.; p. 17.

As time goes on, developmental tasks for individuals evolve, and tasks for the whole family change. For example, as two individuals form themselves into a couple, the family task centers more on building intimacy. Later, if there are children, when the children become adolescents, the family task will center more on ensuring independence and autonomy. Since family challenges vary according to the developmental stage of the family, identifying the life cycle stage helps healthcare practitioners to refine their family-oriented questions.

Minh's life cycle stage is the family with adolescents. Bich's life cycle stage is the graying of the family. Minh and Tam would be described as the "sandwich generation", being in the middle of two life cycle stages. Important tasks are to provide Linh with the necessary personal and academic resources so that his path in life will be a healthy and happy one. Important tasks for Bich are to maintain her functioning as her body declines, to adapt to the loss of her husband, and to prepare for her eventual death. Minh's healthcare practitioner knew Tam from their work together with the community youth organization. She approached Minh about bringing family members to a visit to discuss how the medical system could better support Minh and her family.

CONDUCTING A FAMILY CONFERENCE

Our guide for a family conference describes a process whereby the healthcare practitioner collaborates with the family to set specific healthcare goals, and then identifies a means of reaching these goals. The conference draws on the family's resources to establish a collaborative plan involving the patient, her family, and the healthcare system.[9–15]

Pre-conference

When preparing for a family conference, the healthcare practitioner and the patient need to be clear about the following:

1 Articulate the goal(s) of the family conference: The goal for the family meeting is to strengthen each family member's individual abilities to act in ways that will promote family health and to explore how the health system can better support the patient and their family. *The practitioner suggested to Minh that they meet to discuss the recent changes in the family, their impact on Minh's health, and available resources.*

2 Negotiate who will attend and why: *The practitioner and Minh decided to include Tam and Bich at the next visit, and perhaps to include Linh at a subsequent visit.*

3 Reassure the patient about confidentiality, and establish an acceptable range of topics for the conference: *The healthcare practitioner and Minh discussed whether it would be acceptable to talk about Tam's drinking. They decided together that if he raised the subject, they would all talk about it, but if he didn't raise it, they would try to discuss it at a future visit.*

4 Consider the primary causes of the problem(s) and strategize about how to confirm or refute these hypotheses. Include specific questions, observations, or tasks that will facilitate data gathering and help to test the hypotheses. *The practitioner wanted to know what each family member thought had caused Minh's headaches and fatigue, how Tam was feeling about his retirement, and what was most important for their family at this point in time.* Consider alternative hypotheses during the meeting, and strategies for testing new theories. With a particularly complicated family, consider asking a colleague, especially one with mental health training, to join you in conducting the conference.

The family conference

The family conference can be divided into five phases that generally occur in sequence:

1 Greet the family members.
2 Clarify and further articulate the goals.
3 Discuss the challenges to success.
4 Acknowledge previous successes and current means of success.
5 Make a plan.[1]

Each phase can take between 2 and 10 minutes, depending on whether the healthcare practitioner has met the family members before, on family members' conversational abilities, and on the degree of conflict.

Phase 1: Greeting

Build rapport and help family members to feel at ease in the setting of the conference. Avoid premature attempts to solve the problems by respectfully deferring that important process until after you have had a chance to greet everyone. Briefly converse with each family member about information that is easy to discuss. Remain positive and affirming, making interested comments. *In response to how he was feeling about his retirement, Tam said that it was much more difficult than he had imagined. He then described his work in community politics and the local youth group. The practitioner commented on how lucky the community was to have Tam's managerial talents to apply to community projects.*

Respect the family hierarchy and pay special attention to those whom you have just met or who need extra efforts to make them feel included. *The practitioner has to pay special attention to Bich, who he had never met and who needed to be drawn into the conversation.*

Attend to both verbal and non-verbal behavior, and adapt your style, tone, posture, and vocabulary to fit with the family. Express your gratitude for everyone's commitment to making the family situation better, and acknowledge the sacrifices that family members may have had to make to attend the conference.

Phase 2: Articulate the goals

Ask about each family member's goals. Tam wanted information about his wife's illnesses and how to prevent her increasing disability. Minh was concerned about Tam's health, his weight loss, and the abdominal pains that were waking him up in the morning. Bich was worried about the lack of recognition of all that Minh did in the home.

Rephrase the goals in positive, mutually agreed terms. The healthcare practitioner may need to add his or her own goals. If there are a large number of goals, prioritize them. *Minh and Tam accepted the practitioner's proposal to address Minh's condition in detail and only briefly discuss Tam's condition. A full work-up for Tam could be addressed at another visit.*

Note any conflicting goals.

Phase 3: Discuss the challenges to success

Exchange meaningful information with the family. Acknowledge changes in the family system that influence and are influenced by the presenting concern.

1   Encourage everyone to share their perspective. *After sharing information about the medical aspects of Minh's issues, the practitioner talked about the stresses that were affecting her health. She then asked the family members to say what they thought had impacted on Minh's health.*

2   If appropriate, include the views of others outside the family (e.g., friends, neighbors, folk healers) by asking questions such as *"Who has given you advice about this problem?"*

3   Note recent events that could impact on the issue of concern, such as moves, illness, death, occupational shifts, marriages, divorces, or births.

4   Observe the family process and be prepared to interrupt with phrases such as *"I think that's really important, and I'd like to get back to that, but right now I would like to hear from . . . or . . . about . . ."*

5   Recognize, explicitly acknowledge, and respond to any emotions that are expressed. For example, *"Minh, I can see how sad you are"* or *"Tam, I can imagine how disappointed and frustrated you must be."*

6   Clearly express understanding, but also be clear that understanding does not necessarily imply agreement. Make sure that each person expresses their own

point of view. *The healthcare practitioner needed to actively interrupt Tam to allow Bich to share her perspective. As the family meeting unfolded, Tam admitted to spending many hours drinking with his buddies over lunch. He knew that this was not healthy for him or his family, but he didn't know what else he could do. He had begun drinking daily and noticed that his increased drinking was making him feel more and more isolated from his family. Bich finally commented on her concern for the emotional safety of Minh, and stared at Tam.*

7 Remain as detached and "objective" as possible. *In response to Bich's comment, the practitioner asked what she meant. Tam then admitted that he was losing control of his temper. He had been feeling "not himself" since his retirement, and was doing things that he would never have dreamed of doing previously – hitting the walls, throwing things, and most recently physically shaking Minh when he was upset. All of the family members agreed that this was new behavior for Tam, and that Linh and the children had never seen this behavior before. The practitioner acknowledged the stresses that Tam was experiencing, and stated that it was not a healthy situation. No one should be treated that way, and there was help available for Tam and his family. When he was asked what was most important to him at this time, Tam said Minh and his family. He was ready to do anything he could to make things better for them.*

8 Provide ample time for questions towards the end of the conference. *Surprisingly, Tam asked if the practitioner could provide any help for him to stop drinking. He had experienced problems with drinking when he was young, but when he started his military career his drinking problems diminished. This provided a clue to Tam's recovery. He admitted that he needed to be redirected away from alcohol-related activities and to feel that he was contributing to his family and the community.*

Phase 4: Acknowledge previous successes and current means of success

Recognize the available resources that can be brought to bear on the issue(s) of concern.

1 Identify family resources and strengths. Ask family members to point out the strengths that they see in themselves, in each other and in overall family functioning.[1] This is a powerful exercise because it is supportive, and because it can reduce the temptation to demand unnecessary or less effective services outside the family. Develop a list of family members and friends who are available to the patient. In a stressed family, the healthcare practitioner may need to help with this task. *The practitioner pointed out the love and commitment of Bich, Minh, and Tam to one another, and Tam's honesty and willingness to take responsibility for his contributions to the problems and the solutions. Tam's prognosis was good if he could stop or at least control his drinking, particularly given that his behaviors were relatively new.*

2 Identify health resources and healers outside the family (*see* Chapter 6). Help family members to specify clearly their expectations of service practitioners. *Bich was already established with the nephrologist in the district health center, but saw the physician infrequently, because the family had to borrow a car and*

drive the two-hour journey to the kidney specialist's office. Ensure that there are accurate expectations with regard to what services can be provided. *The practitioner explained what medical services she and her team could provide at the local level for Bich and for Tam. She pointed out that Tam's stomach problems could be related to his drinking. She discussed setting up an individual visit with Tam to work up the stomach pain.*

3 Identify other resources outside the family, including women's groups, religious organizations, health outreach workers, and other community groups available to support the patient and/or their family. *The healthcare practitioner would go into more detail at Tam's next medical visit about alcohol treatment options (rehabilitation, medication, support groups), depending on Tam's ability to stop or control his drinking between visits.*

Phase 5: Make a plan

1 Explicitly outline a mutually agreed upon treatment plan and define each person's role in carrying out the plan. *Tam was willing to cut down on his drinking and to explore ways to expand his contribution to his home or the community. He would also try counting to 10 before addressing his frustrations, and would walk away if he felt the urge to physically act out his anger. Minh was willing to comment on the good things that Tam was doing, and to involve him in more of the decisions that were made in the home. Bich was willing to work at improving her blood sugar levels, in order to have more energy to help around the house.*

2 Emphasize the areas that represent common ground, and negotiate compromises where necessary. If conflict remains, make a plan for a future means of resolving conflict.

3 Draw up a health contract with the family that defines who is going to do what and within what time frame. The health contract is a verbal or written summary that outlines:
— what each family member will do
— what the practitioner will do
— referrals
— follow-up appointment.[1]

This case illustrates how a healthcare practitioner might bring a family together to discuss a health-related issue. The practitioner was able to lead a family discussion in which family members were willing to address the very sensitive issues of alcohol abuse and domestic violence. In this family meeting, Tam was willing to admit his difficulties and to work with the healthcare practitioner and the family to remedy his problems. Often, however, domestic violence is much more hidden and resistant to change.[16,17] If Tam had not mentioned the abuse, the practitioner would not have raised the subject for discussion or encouraged Minh to raise it at the meeting. This could have placed Minh in greater danger by discussing the violence during the family conference, and risked causing more anger in the abusive person.

Because of the hidden nature of domestic violence, the use of midwives and healthcare workers or health promoters from within the community can be very helpful in identifying and assisting these women and their families. One in three women worldwide will suffer from some form of violence in their lifetime. Domestic violence, described as an escalating pattern of abuse, has lifelong negative consequences for the physical and mental health of the person being abused, and for children who witness the abuse. Studies have shown that around 70% of men who abuse their spouse or partner also abuse their children.[16] Women who have been abused tend to visit healthcare practitioners more frequently than those who have not been abused.[17] Additional training and resources to enable healthcare practitioners to address domestic violence are listed below.

CONCLUSION

Most primary care practitioners can be competent mediators within the family as a result of targeted skill building and focused reflection on family dynamics. A healthcare practitioner who knows the family members and how they function together has the ability to negotiate the patient's care and help the whole family. For if they do not address family issues such as those of Minh and Tam, who will? It is essential to develop good family interviewing skills that allow a healthcare practitioner to direct discussions so that the maximum amount of information can be shared clearly in the shortest amount of time. Working with families is an efficient and responsible way to provide healthcare. In Minh's case, the family meeting was an intervention that changed the course of their family functioning for the better.

KEY RESOURCES

- McDaniel S, Campbell T, Hepworth J, *et al. Family-Oriented Primary Care.* 2nd ed. New York: Springer; 2005.
- **Family Violence Prevention Fund.** *Maternal Health and Safety in a Multicultural Context: toolkit for, rural healthcare providers and advocates*; http://endabuse.org/content/features/detail/813/ (accessed 18 May 2009).
- **World Health Organization.** *Violence Against Women and Achieving the Millennium Development Goals*; www.who.int/gender/documents/MDGs&VAWSept05.pdf (accessed 18 May 2009).

REFERENCES

1 McDaniel S, Campbell T, Hepworth J, *et al. Family-Oriented Primary Care.* 2nd ed. New York: Springer; 2005.
2 McGoldrick M, Gerson R. *Genograms in Family Assessment.* New York: WW Norton; 1985.
3 Jolly W, Froom J, Rosen M. The genogram. *J Fam Pract.* 1980; **2**: 251–5.
4 McGoldrick M, Giordano J, Pearce J. *Ethnicity and Family Therapy.* New York: Guilford Press; 1996.
5 Carter B, McGoldrick M. *The Changing Family Life Cycle: a framework for family therapy.* 2nd ed. Lebanon, IN: Prentice Hall College Division; 1989.
6 Duvall EM. *Marriage and Family Development.* Philadelphia, PA: Lippincott; 1977.

7 Hill R. *Family Development in Three Generations*. Cambridge, MA: Schenkman; 1970.

8 Combrinck-Graham L. A developmental model for family systems. *Fam Process*. 1985; **24**: 139.

9 Meyer D, Schneid J, Craigie FC. Family conferences: reasons, levels of involvement and perceived usefulness. *J Fam Pract*. 1989; **29**: 401–5.

10 Kushner K, Meyer D, Hansen JP. Patients' attitudes toward health care provider involvement in family conferences. *J Fam Pract*. 1989; **28**: 73–8.

11 Kushner K, Meyer D, Hansen M, *et al.* What do patients want? *J Fam Pract*. 1986; **23**: 463–7.

12 Haley J. *Problem-Solving Therapy*. San Francisco, CA: Jossey-Bass; 1987.

13 Weber T, McKeever J, McDaniel S. A beginner's guide to the problem-oriented first family interview. *Fam Process*. 1985; **24**: 357–64.

14 Talbot Y. *Families: the "how." The family in family medicine: graduate curriculum and teaching strategies*. Leewood, KS: Society of Teachers of Family Medicine; 1981.

15 McDaniel S, Campbell T, Wynne L, *et al.* Family systems consultation: opportunities for teaching in family medicine. *Fam Syst Med*. 1987; **6**: 391–403.

16 Bowker A, McFerron A. On the relationship between wife beating and child abuse. In: Yilo K, Bogard M (eds) *Feminist Perspectives on Wife Abuse*. Beverly Hills, CA: Sage; 1988.

17 Saunders DG, Hamberher K, Hovey M. Indicators of woman abuse based on chart review at a family practice center. *Arch Fam Med*. 1993; **2**: 537–43.

CHAPTER 6

Social and cultural influences

Daniel L Meyer, Julie M Schirmer and Nguyen Minh Tam

CASE SCENARIO 1

Deqa Ashid is a 19-year-old Somali mother who has been experiencing fatigue, decreased energy, and difficulties sleeping and eating since the birth of her 6-week-old daughter. Her daughter had been born in the family hut by strapping a rope around the center ridge pole which Deqa grabbed to assist in the delivery. Her baby was delivered into a small, blanketed pit that she and her husband had carefully carved out of the earth. She was lucky to have a traditional birth attendant from a nearby village in attendance. She, her husband and her husband's brother's family are nomads, continually moving together across the plains of northern Somalia, following the migration of their camels and cattle to the seasonal sources of food and water.

CASE SCENARIO 2

Arwalla Mohammud is an 18-year-old Somali mother of three children, who has been fatigued and in constant anxiety since the birth of her 8-week-old son. She wakes him every two hours, day and night, to feed him. She is extremely concerned that he is not getting enough to eat, and she secretly fears that her breast milk is not good enough for the baby. She has begun arguing with her mother, aunts, and sisters, as she feels that they don't understand what she is going through and that they don't have confidence in her ability to care for her baby. She is not sleeping, has lost weight, and has deep circles under her eyes. Her mother and sisters are concerned about the changes in her mood and her behaviors, and in how she has been relating to them since her son was born. So they took her to the doctor when the baby was 3 weeks old. They live in Somalia's capital city, where there are doctors in government-run and private outpatient clinics.

INTRODUCTION

This chapter reviews the basic cultural theories, concepts, attitudes, knowledge, and skills that must be considered when providing primary healthcare. General principles for developing and delivering culturally sensitive care are discussed in relation to the two case scenarios described above. Community-oriented primary care principles are outlined to help primary care practitioners to address behavioral and mental health issues in the communities in which they serve. The final section provides advice on how healthcare practitioners can prepare to work in cultures different from their own. The skills and techniques addressed in this chapter apply to practitioner–patient encounters within pluralistic, heterogeneous societies where refugees and immigrants are plentiful. They also apply to patient, teaching, or consulting encounters where healthcare practitioners are practicing in another country.

We admit to the difficulties of trying to distill a very complex construct such as culture into a set of skills and techniques that might lead a healthcare practitioner to cultural competence or expertise. These constructs and strategies are intended to be used as beginning steps to continually improve healthcare practitioners' care of patients and communities.

THE IMPORTANCE OF CULTURE

Cultural beliefs and practices exert powerful and often unrecognized influences on patients' health and well-being, as well as on their knowledge and use of available healers. The Merriam-Webster Dictionary Online (2009) defines culture as follows:

> 5b: the customary beliefs, social forms, and material traits of a racial, religious, or social group; also 5c: the characteristic features of everyday existence (as diversions or a way of life) shared by people in a place or time . . . the set of shared attitudes, values, goals, and practices that characterizes an institution or organization, also 5d: the set of values, conventions, or social practices associated with a particular field, activity, or societal characteristic.[1]

This definition, of course, applies worldwide.

Indeed, even within a single culture, worldviews of healthcare practitioners, patients, and health systems can be starkly different and can easily complicate a treatment encounter. Specifically, patients' beliefs about the causes and treatments of their symptoms, drawn from their culture, can generate expectations and judgments about healthcare practitioners' examination skills and treatment advice. Practitioners' beliefs that evidence-based treatments are the best medicine can be in direct conflict with their patients' beliefs about treatment. Health systems beliefs about what is important to healthcare become implemented through staffing patterns, management structure, and reimbursement policies. For example, in the USA, reimbursement parity, as in providing the same payment for mental health disorders as for physical health disorders, has been an ongoing struggle.

Culture has become more and more important as countries have become increasingly interconnected. Immigrants represent approximately 12% of the total US population,[2] 18% of the Canadian population, and 9% of the UK population.[3] Since 1983, the USA has accepted nearly 2 million refugees who have settled in 331 predominantly metropolitan areas.[4] Many of these communities are fairly homogeneous, such as the Minneapolis area, which has a high concentration of people from South-East Asia. This differs from the New England states, where immigrants from a wide range of cultures live in the same communities.[4] For example, over 50 different languages are spoken in the schools and hospitals of Portland, Maine.[5]

Cultural beliefs, norms, and values can be viewed from a national perspective (shared across the country as a whole), from a regional perspective (taking into consideration differences in ethnicity, language, or religion), or taking into consideration differences in gender, generations (both within families and across communities), or social class (social, educational, and occupational characteristics and assumptions). Because of this cultural diversity, it is extremely important not to stereotype people on the basis of their ethnicity or culture, or to see every patient issue as specifically culturally determined (*see* the case description on page 12 in Chapter 1).

INSIDER VERSUS OUTSIDER PERSPECTIVES
Medical anthropology and medical sociology are fields of study concerned with cultural issues and how they relate to health and healthcare.[6] Among the more important concepts in these fields of study is that of "insider" versus "outsider" perspectives when considering culture. Both perspectives play a significant role in developing clinical assessments and plans that will work within the cultural context of a medical encounter. Insiders (usually the patients) have learned the culture from within and, when asked, can be important sources of insight into local knowledge, beliefs, and behavior. Outsiders (usually the healthcare practitioners) bring other cultural experiences and biases to the encounter, and unless they are unusually inquisitive and non-judgmental, they may be unaware of the contradictions between the two perspectives.

Anthropologists use an "ethnographic" approach to better understand the insider perspective of a given group of people. An ethnographer goes into a foreign country, learns the language, and lives, breathes, and works among the people in order to better understand their social, moral, and religious views and practices. To apply an ethnographic approach to patient care, healthcare practitioners must begin to:

1 learn about common local health beliefs and practices of their patients
2 understand how the local culture's family structures, values, and everyday activities shape how behavioral interventions might work in the local context
3 be aware of other professional and lay practitioners of healthcare and healing.

In the first scenario, Deqa's daughter was born 2 months premature. Immediately after the delivery, the birth attendant was concerned that the baby would not survive for more than a few days. The baby finally began to gain weight and became responsive and lively. During the first couple of weeks, Deqa's husband and family had read the Qur'an nightly in the hut to pray to God for her and her baby's health. They stopped, once they saw that the baby was thriving. They would never have considered going to the birth attendant or any other healthcare practitioner, particularly since they lived in such a barren part of the country, with minimal health resources. The family believed that if this was Deqa's or her baby's time to die, then they would provide a peaceful and Godly presence to usher them into the next life. They also thought that, due to their circumstances, there was nothing they could do to improve their health.

Clearly, this family held a set of beliefs that was unlikely to be shared by an "outsider."

DISEASE VERSUS ILLNESS

A second set of important cultural concepts is "disease" versus "illness." As described in Chapter 2, disease is generally a Western medical definition with an "objective" reproducible measurement, such as a high blood glucose reading or a physical finding. Clearly, this is the "outsider's" perspective. Illness, on the other hand, is the patient's ("insider's") experience (i.e. what they are feeling or experiencing, and how this is affecting their life). Even within a Western medical context, there can be little or no correlation between these two. Examples of disease findings in the absence of perceived illness include high blood pressure readings during screening, early stages of HIV infection, etc. Examples of illness in the absence of "medical" disease findings include psychosomatic complaints and other unexplained symptoms (see Chapter 3).

Although they did not initially perceive themselves as having a disease or an illness, Deqa and Arwalla were both experiencing depression, more specifically postpartum depression, named for its occurrence immediately after the birth of their babies. Postpartum depression affects 10–15% of women in developed countries, and is estimated to have even higher rates in developing countries.[7]

Studies have shown that postpartum depression can have negative consequences for mothers and infants which may last into adulthood. It is associated with suboptimal breastfeeding,[8] delays in seeking help for serious childhood illnesses,[9] infant malnutrition,[10,11] and impaired mental and motor development.[12,13] Because of these negative consequences it is vitally important for healthcare practitioners to screen for and address the mother's postpartum depression or any other mental health issues during and after pregnancy. Treatment includes increased social support, counseling, or medication if the depression is severely affecting the functioning of the mother (see Chapters 7 and 8).

The issues related to disease and illness can become even more complex outside the Western medical context. Anthropologists have identified "culturally defined syndromes" as insiders' experience of signs and symptoms that are not part of Western interpretations.[6] Common examples are the "ataque de nervios," neurasthenia (*see* Chapter 3), and "susto" or shock in Mexican cultures. These have no Western counterparts, and may be perceived by outsiders as superstition.[14] Furthermore, symptoms of depression and anxiety are not typically regarded as illnesses in most of the developing world, and therefore would not motivate people affected by them to access healthcare. Depression and anxiety could well be considered culturally defined syndromes of the developed world, by many living in rural Asia, Africa, or the Middle East.

In the second, urban scenario, Arwalla's family took her to a doctor, who thought that she was experiencing postpartum depression. He pointed out that she was stressed and burdened. After making sure that she and the baby were safe, he told the family that he was concerned about her decreased functioning and that she would benefit from medication. Arwalla's mother and aunt would have none of that. They refused to go to the pharmacy to collect the recommended medication, and told Arwalla not to take the medication. They had hoped that the doctor would find some physical reason for her symptoms and would suggest a shot or some other quick remedy.

As these cases illustrate, although the mothers in these scenarios are both from Somalia, their lives, beliefs, and access to healthcare resources are extremely different.

ALTERNATIVE WAYS OF CONCEPTUALIZING HEALTH AND CARE

A useful area of anthropological inquiry has been cross-cultural explorations of explanatory approaches to disease causation and interventions. Primary care practitioners need to be sensitive to patients' perceptions of disease and illness causation,[15] especially when seeing patients in communities other than the practitioner's own. Scrimshaw provides examples across nine categories of disease causation (*see* Table 6.1). As with the indigenous medical system, healthcare practitioners must be aware of, and even make use of, such explanatory belief systems. It is particularly important to understand a culture's explanatory models and definitions of behavioral disorders, because these may be very different from the Western medical traditions.

TABLE 6.1 Types of cultural explanations of disease causation

Body balance:	Supernatural:
Temperature: hot or cold	Bewitching
Energy	Demons
Blood: loss of blood; properties of blood	Spirit possession
reflecting imbalance; pollution from	Evil eye
menstruation	Offending God or gods
Emotional:	Soul loss
Fright	Behavior in a past life
Sorrow	**Food:**
Envy	Properties: hot, cold, heavy, light
Stress	Spoiled foods
Weather:	Dirty foods
Winds	Sweets
Change of weather	Raw foods
Seasonal imbalance	Combining the "wrong" foods
Vectors or organisms:	Mud
Worms	**Sexual:**
Flies	Sex with a forbidden person
Parasites	Overindulgence in sex
Germs	Masturbation
	Heredity
	Old age

Reprinted with permission from Scrimshaw SC. Culture, behavior, and health. In: Merson MH, Black RE, Mills AJ (eds) *International Public Health: diseases, programs, systems, and policies.* Sudbury, MA: Jones and Bartlett; 2001. p. 58.

Patients' beliefs about disease causation help to guide their choice of healers. In many rural parts of the world, folk healers provide treatments that are more congruent with patients' health beliefs, are located much closer to patients, and are usually less costly than the professional healers listed in Table 6.2.[15] When entering different cultural contexts, healthcare practitioners should be aware of these local healing resources, and should reach out to them to better understand their beliefs and practices.

TABLE 6.2 Categories of "healers"

Popular healers:

Self-treatment by patients, families, and friends

Folk healers:

Midwives	Sorcerers
Shamans	Priests
Spiritualists	Medicine men and women
Witches	Ayurvedic practitioners
Herbalists	Injectionists
Birth attendants	

Professional healers:

Doctors	Dentists
Nurse midwives	Pharmacists
Nurses	Acupuncturists
Pharmacists	Traditional medicine doctors
Barefoot doctors	

Adapted from Kleinman A. *Patients and Healers in the Context of Culture: an exploration of the borderland between anthropology, medicine, and psychiatry.* Berkeley, CA: University of California Press; 1980.

Integrative or alternative medicine is a relatively new concept that has been receiving increasing attention in Western medicine, and has direct application when addressing cultural aspects of care. Integrative medicine joins medical therapies and complementary, alternative medical therapies for which there is strong evidence of efficacy and safety.[16] It acknowledges and formally incorporates into care resources and practitioners beyond the traditional Western healthcare delivery system that is found in resource-rich countries.

Deqa's family became very concerned about her weight loss and decreased functioning. Despite the arguments of Deqa's husband to the contrary, Deqa's sister-in-law convinced him to let her take Deqa and her daughter to the home of Deqa's parents in a small village two days' journey away. The village birth attendant had special training in assessing depression and counseling new mothers. She visited Deqa twice a week during her 2-month stay at her parents' home. The attendant never used the term "depression" when talking with Deqa, but used the term "stress" and other words that Deqa herself used when talking about her condition. She used cognitive therapy principles to help Deqa to identify thoughts that were contributing to her depression and reframe them in ways that would improve her mental health (*see* Table 6.3). Because she responded well to the counseling, medication was not needed to return her to her previous level of functioning and back to her husband.

TABLE 6.3 Cultural beliefs about perinatal issues that could be harmful to maternal and child health

Existing belief	Potential "reframing" suggestions
My baby will get ill, it's kismet (fate).	There are many things that can be done to increase my chances of having a healthy baby, such as vaccines, vitamins, a healthy diet, and seeing my healthcare practitioner.
Girls need less attention and care than boys.	All infants need to be cared for, played with, and loved.
Being ill is my fate (feeding into an illness–hopelessness cycle).	I can do a number of things to increase the health of myself and my baby.
I am unwell because of the effects of a spell from an evil person or spirit. I will feel better only after the spell is broken.	I can take positive action and use traditional help. Modern and traditional care can both be pursued for best results.
Illness is a punishment for my deeds.	I can focus on what is good in my life and on what I can do.
I have too many problems. Looking after my own health is a low priority.	If one is not healthy, even small problems look big. If I am healthy, I can give full attention to my children.
My husband doesn't understand. If I talk to him it will create further conflict.	Although my husband and I have differences, we must talk about our child's welfare.
I don't deserve to get well.	Despite my difficulties, I have to try to decrease my tension and anxiety for my baby.

Adapted from Rahman A. Challenges and opportunities in developing a psychological intervention for perinatal depression in rural Pakistan – a multi-method study. *Arch Womens Ment Health*. 2007:**10**: 213.

In Arwalla's case, her husband was increasingly concerned about her increased irritability, pacing at night, lack of sleep, and decreased functioning at home. He and his mother convinced Arwalla that the doctor knew what he was doing. She began to take the medication. Within a couple of days her sleep and her mood had improved. She began to slowly regain her strength to go grocery shopping, to start taking care of chores around the home, and to visit friends and family.

As the situations of Deqa and Arwalla show, families can either inhibit or facilitate patients' willingness to accept Western medicine's diagnosis and treatment.

ETHNOCENTRISM

A final anthropological concept of importance is "ethnocentrism", or the implicit assumption that one's culture of origin, to the exclusion of others, has the only correct worldview. Ethnocentrism can negatively influence not only the practitioner's judgment about what is right or wrong, but also the patient's point of view.

Practitioners working in international settings therefore need to keep this potential hazard in mind.

> Arwalla's son was delivered in a university hospital with an obstetrician in attendance. Her mother, aunts, and sisters cleaned, shopped, cooked, and cared for her for 40 days after the birth of her son, in accordance with the custom called *Afartan Bax*. The belief is that new mothers and babies should not go outside the home during the first 40 days, as this is when they need to be healed and are extremely vulnerable to disease and evil spirits.

Thus, despite a Western-style delivery, cultural beliefs led the family to keep the mother in seclusion, making it impossible for a physician to see her and the baby for follow-up until the end of the 40-day period. Unless there was an outreach system, whereby trained health workers visited patients in their homes, Arwalla and her baby would not receive any healthcare until the 40-day period was over.

In summary, patients need to be approached within the framework of their culture. Their values, beliefs, and assumptions guide the actions of both patient and physician. Thus it is important to understand the patient's family, work, and community contexts. At the level of the individual encounter, physicians need to know what the patient thinks is causing their problem or symptom, what the symptom means to the patient (e.g. short-term, chronic, or trivial problem, fatal condition), what has already been tried, and what their expectations are for the outcome of the individual encounter itself (medication, acupuncture, referral, or something else). Each of these factors is shaped by the cultural context of the patient. Women will act and think differently from men, one religious tradition will be contrary to another, and other cultural divisions such as age, racial subgroups, etc. will each have their own varying effects.

As each of the chapters in this text is approached by the reader, specific cultural influences should be considered. Family systems vary across cultures. For example, how many generations typically live in the same dwelling? Do specific family members make the health decisions? How do the roles and responsibilities of parents and children change across the life cycle?

Behavioral and psychiatric definitions and diagnoses are likely to differ according to the culture. For example, the above cases clearly illustrate that depression is not recognized or acknowledged by Deqa, Arwalla, or their families as an "illness" or "disease" that needs medical attention. It can be very important for practitioners to listen to the words patients use to describe their problem and to use those words as much as possible when diagnosing and treating the problem. In addition, behavioral health practitioners and medications are not available in some settings.

The role of a healthcare practitioner varies across cultures, from respected healthcare practitioner to healer of last resort or point of entry into specialty care. Finally, how do the behavioral assessment and intervention approaches and techniques described in this text fit into the existing culture? Some questions or issues may be taboo. What are the resources available – Western or "indigenous" – to address them? In Deqa's case, she was lucky to have a birth attendant assist with the birth of her child, given the isolated lifestyle of this family. The outcome would have been much graver if her sister-in-law had not convinced Deqa's husband that she needed to return to her parents' home.

COMMUNITY-ORIENTED PRIMARY CARE

Community-oriented primary care (COPC) is a systematic way for primary care practitioners to identify and address the health needs of a given population. It helps to improve practitioners' understanding of the health beliefs and needs of people in a particular community, and it also improves community members' understanding of primary healthcare. In the USA, Community Health Centers, the Indian Health Service, and Health Maintenance Organizations have long been using COPC strategies to plan care for entire communities. In the developing world, primary care projects have used COPC principles to address issues such as infant mortality, use of safe drinking water, and mental health needs.[17,18]

The core steps of the COPC process are as follows:

1 defining a population
2 assessing the health needs of the population
3 developing a program to meet the health needs of that population
4 evaluating the results.[17]

The population can be as extensive as all persons living in a geographically defined area, or as restricted as all people with depression in a given primary care practice.

A primary care project in the District of Machakos, Kenya, demonstrates how some of the COPC strategies are applied to entire communities.[18] The purpose of the project was to recruit and train community health workers (CHWs) to help to identify and then address the health needs in their communities.

Prior to going into the district, the project coordinator used census data, government documents, informant interviews, and textbooks to help to *define the community*. He sought to understand the people, their history, how they worked and lived, their current issues, and formal and informal leaders. The coordinator involved community leaders from the very beginning. He began to *assess health needs* by meeting with leaders to get their perspective on health needs and to ask for their help with the project. The chiefs, government health officials, and women's group leaders identified and chose the CHWs for their communities.

The CHW training was very participatory and was based on what the CHWs thought were the most important community health problems (enhanced by information from previous research and interviews with community leaders), and on what they knew about factors that contributed to sickness and health. The CHWs conducted focus groups in their communities, asking similar questions.

Overall district problems included drought, famine, malnutrition, and increased modernization, which drew the men to the cities, leaving the women primarily responsible for caring for their homes and raising the children. Infant and child mortality rates in the district were very high. Several of the popular and folk beliefs about and treatments for malnutrition were potentially dangerous, as they postponed or prevented treatment that could save children's lives. The CHWs were taught to neither encourage nor discourage traditional health beliefs and treatments, as they themselves were probably biased and likely to have participated in the practices. Moreover, the folk healers were likely to be community leaders. The CHWs would also lose credibility if they returned to their communities and told everyone that they did everything wrong.

The CHWs were instructed in nutrition and sanitation practices for prevention, and were taught how to use rehydration solution to treat dehydration. They then took this new knowledge and these new skills back to their communities (*program to meet the needs of the population*). The CHWs gained credibility as a result of their treatment successes, and infant and child mortality rates improved (*evaluation of results*).

GENERAL PRINCIPLES OF CULTURALLY SENSITIVE HEALTHCARE

Culturally sensitive practice guidelines have been developed for the training of healthcare professionals. It is helpful to know the community's cultural perspective on medicine and health, the epidemiology of the area, and something of the language. Equally important is an attitude of cultural humility – an honest stance of "not knowing" the multiple factors of patients' lives, culture, or community. Core attitudes and knowledge areas have been developed to guide culturally sensitive practices for primary healthcare practitioners (*see* Tables 6.4 and 6.5).

TABLE 6.4 Attitudes for culturally sensitive healthcare

1	Awareness of socio-cultural factors that contribute to health
2	Acceptance of the practitioner's responsibility to understand the cultural dimensions of their patients and the communities in which they practice
3	Appreciation of the heterogeneity of principles within and across cultural groups
4	Recognition of personal biases and reactions to people from other groups
5	Awareness of one's own personal cultural values and how they affect patient care
6	Recognition of historical, political, economic, and environmental forces on healthcare
7	Respect for and tolerance of difference

Abbreviated from Like R, Steiner RP, Rubel A. STFM Core Curriculum Guidelines: recommended core curriculum guidelines on culturally sensitive and competent health care, p. 292; http://stfm.org/corep.html (accessed 14 January 2009).

TABLE 6.5 Knowledge base for culturally sensitive healthcare

I. Cultural perspective on medicine and public health
    A. Health-seeking and illness behaviors of patients
    B. Distinction between disease and illness
    C. Family and personal health- and illness-related beliefs, attitudes, customs, and values
    D. Socio-cultural risk factors and potential interventions

I. Cultural perspective on medicine and public health

    E. Use of various health sectors (indigenous, pluralistic, and Western)

    F. Access and barriers to care

II. Cultural epidemiology

    A. Clinical problems related to national health promotion and disease prevention

    B. Problems related to high morbidity and mortality rates

    C. Problems related to individual and family life cycle and major life events

    D. Problems related to migration and intergenerational conflicts

    E. Problems related to "folk" illnesses

Abbreviated from Like R, Steiner RP, Rubel A. STFM Core Curriculum Guidelines: recommended core curriculum guidelines on culturally sensitive and competent health care, p. 293; http://stfm.org/corep.html (accessed 14 January 2009).

The skills that are required for culturally sensitive healthcare are listed in Table 6.6. In the care of the mothers described in the two scenarios in this chapter, these skills were essential.

TABLE 6.6 Skills for culturally sensitive healthcare

1	Form and maintain a therapeutic alliance.
2	Recognize and respond appropriately to verbal and non-verbal communication.
3	Obtain medical and psychosocial histories and perform a culturally sensitive exam.
4	Use the biopsychosocial model in disease prevention/health promotion, interpret clinical data, and problem-solve around illnesses.
5	Prescribe culturally sensitive medication and treatment.
6	Understand by eliciting the patient's explanatory models, including their understanding of illness and their treatment expectations.
7	Explore psychosocial context of patients (not a patient visit).
8	Work with family and community members.
9	Work with other health professionals.
10	Work with lay and indigenous healers when appropriate.
11	Identify how the practitioner's cultural values, assumptions, and beliefs affect patient care and decision making.

Abbreviated from Like R, Steiner RP, Rubel A. STFM Core Curriculum Guidelines: recommended core curriculum guidelines on culturally sensitive and competent health care, p. 294; http://stfm.org/corep.html (accessed 14 January 2009).

PREPARING TO WORK IN HEALTHCARE SETTINGS IN A DIFFERENT CULTURE

There are multiple strategies to prepare one for healthcare practice in a community different from one's own. High-speed Internet connections provide immediate access to information about medical epidemiology and cultural perspectives on medicine and public health. For example, during the preparation of this chapter, Internet searches identified links to sites that described aspects of "generic" Vietnamese culture, as well as sub-cultural groups within it. An Internet-based article on the culture and farming of the northern mountain region of Vietnam identified three main ethnic groups and several small groups, each with varying beliefs and practices.[19] The WHO Atlas Project provides information on how healthcare systems are structured and on the availability of medical and behavioral health practitioners in most countries of the world.[20] The US Peace Corps offers online training manuals for volunteers who work in the more than 74 developing countries around the world.[21] A 2007 article on global health curriculum lists multiple Internet-based resources that can help to prepare the practitioner for work in healthcare overseas.[22]

"Cultural informants" can provide insights about patients' beliefs, health-seeking behaviors, and medical systems before or during work in a new community. Multiple sources from different sectors of a community can deepen an outsider's perspective. However, a word of caution is needed. When applying any of this information one must not assume that, just because patients are from a particular community, they necessarily subscribe to the predominant beliefs and values of the culture. Healthcare practitioners must certainly be aware of the influences of culture on the clinical encounter, but they must also be sensitive to the individual's unique personal thoughts and feelings.

The healthcare practitioners in the above two case scenarios might have been more helpful if they had been aware of what ethnic group the women belonged to, since many different groups can inhabit a particular region. This may be especially relevant if the healthcare practitioner belongs to a different ethnic group, as local history or experience may cause suspicion or distrust on both sides. It is important to keep in mind the fact that not every member of an ethnic group subscribes to group beliefs. The two case scenarios described in this chapter also illustrate the cultural and social differences that are typically found between urban and rural populations.

A number of questions should always be kept in mind. Do gender expectations play a role for either the patient or the practitioner? What do indigenous practitioners use when treating various problems? What beliefs could the patient have about what is causing a problem? What treatments are expected from the Western medical practitioner (injections, pills, X-ray, ultrasound)? Finally, it would be useful to know what patients' role expectations are for care of home and family, and how the health problem is affecting these aspects of their lives. All of these issues can only be addressed when the practitioner has adequate knowledge of and interest in the cultural context of the encounter.

CONCLUSION

Cultural issues need be considered when planning and delivering care. Every clinical encounter occurs within a cultural context that includes community beliefs, professional and patient expectations, local practices, and existing resources. Training and on-site resources exist to assist clinicians as they prepare to deliver care either in their own clinical practices or in international settings.

KEY RESOURCES

- **American Medical Student Association:** a search for international medicine found 225 links; www.amsa.org
- **Global Health Education Consortium:** promotes and facilitates global health education; http://globalhealthedu.org/pages/default.aspx
- **Society of Teachers of Family Medicine (STFM):** provides curriculum guidelines on culturally sensitive and competent care; http://stfm.org/corep. html
- Evert J, Bazemore A, Hixon A, *et al.* Going global: considerations for introducing global health into family medicine training programs. *Fam Med.* 2007; **39**: 659–65; www.stfm.org/fmhub/fm2007/October/Jessica659.pdf
- **WHO Atlas Project:** lists mental health resources for each country worldwide; www.who.int/mental_health/evidence/atlas/en/index.html
- **Peace Corps:** offers online training manuals on what to know before working in 74 different countries; www.peacecorps.gov/index.cfm?shell=learn. wherepc&cid=map

REFERENCES

1 *Merriam-Webster Dictionary Online.* Springfield, MA: Merriam-Webster; 2009; www. merriam-webster.com/dictionary/culture (accessed 16 May 2009).
2 Grieco E. *Immigrant Union Members: numbers and trends*; www.migrationpolicy.org/ pubs/7_Immigrant_Union_Membership.pdf (accessed 17 January 2009).
3 United Nations, Department of Economic and Social Affairs, Population Division. *International Migration 2006*; www.un.org/esa/population/publications/2006Migration_ Chart/2006IttMig_chart.htm (accessed 16 May 2009).
4 Singer A, Wilson JH. *Refugee Resettlement in Metropolitan America.* Washington, DC: The Brookings Institute; 2007; www.migrationinformation.org/Feature/display. cfm?id=585 (accessed 16 May 2009).
5 Valenzuela G. *Demographic Data.* Portland, ME: Portland Public Schools, Multilingual and Multicultural Center; www.portlandschools.org/schools/multilingual/index.html (accessed 28 January 2009).
6 Scrimshaw SC. Culture, behavior, and health. In: Merson MH, Black RE, Mills AJ (eds) *International Public Health: diseases, programs, systems, and policies.* Gaithersburg, MD: Aspen Publishers; 2001. pp. 53–78.
7 O'Hara MW. The nature of postpartum depression disorders. In: Murray L, Cooper PJ (eds) *Postpartum Depression and Child Development.* New York: Guilford Press; 1997. pp. 3–31.
8 Paulson JF, Dauber S, Leiferman JA. Individual and combined effects of postpartum depression in mothers and fathers on parenting behavior. *Pediatrics.* 2006; **118**: 659–68.
9 Chung EK, McCollum KF, Elo IT, *et al.* Maternal depressive symptoms and infant health practices among low-income women. *Pediatrics.* 2004; **113**: 523–9.
10 Patel V, Rahman A, Jacob KS, *et al.* Effect of maternal mental health on infant growth in low-income countries: new evidence from South Asia. *BMJ.* 2004; **328**: 820–23.
11 Rahman A, Lovel H, Bunn J, *et al.* Mothers' mental health and infant growth: a case–control study from Rawalpindi, Pakistan. *Child Care Health Dev.* 2004; **30**: 21–7.
12 Galler JR, Harrison RH, Ramsey F, *et al.* Maternal depressive symptoms affect infant cognitive development in Barbados. *J Child Psychol Psychiatry.* 2000; **41**: 747–57.

13 Galler JR, Ramsey FC, Harrison RH, *et al.* Postpartum maternal moods and infant size predict performance on a national high school entrance examination. *J Child Psychol Psychiatry.* 2004; **45**: 1064–75.

14 Mechanic D. *Medical Sociology: a selective view.* New York: Free Press; 1968.

15 Kleinman A. *Patients and Healers in the Context of Culture: an exploration of the borderland between anthropology, medicine, and psychiatry.* Berkeley, CA: University of California Press; 1980.

16 National Institute for Mental Health, National Center for Complementary and Alternative Therapies. *What is CAM?*; http://nccam.nih.gov/health/whatiscam/overview.htm (accessed 18 January 2009).

17 Nutting P (ed.) *Community-Oriented Primary Care: from principle to practice.* Washington, DC: US Department of Health and Human Services; 1987.

18 Crowley J. *"We Have Done It Ourselves!" A community-based health care program.* Nairobi, Kenya: Medical Department, Kenya Catholic Secretariat; 1987.

19 Vien TD. Culture, environment, and farming systems in Vietnam's northern mountain region. *Southeast Asian Studies.* 2003; **41**: 2180–205.

20 World Health Organization. *Project ATLAS: resources for mental health*; www.who.int/mental_health/evidence/atlas/en/index.html (accessed 29 January 2009).

21 Peace Corps. *Where Do Volunteers Go?*; www.peacecorps.gov/index.cfm?shell=learn.wherepc&cid=map (accessed 18 January 2009).

22 Evert J, Bazemore A, Hixon A, *et al.* Going global: considerations for introducing global health into family medicine training programs. *Fam Med.* 2007; **39**: 659–65.

CHAPTER 7

The management of common mental health concerns in primary care

Jeffrey Stovall, William Ventres, Thich Linh and Le Than Toan

Jemila is an 18-year-old Afghani woman who is brought to see her doctor at the family medicine clinic in a US city by her mother, reporting difficulty sleeping, weakness, and not eating. She states, "My heart is heavy with worry for my brother, who is in the military in Afghanistan. We have not heard from him for 6 months' time." Jemila admits that for the past 6 weeks she has been getting only 3 to 6 hours of sporadic sleep each night. This is affecting her thinking, concentration, mood, and interest in her normal activities. She has had difficulty doing her schoolwork, and has been increasingly late for school, where she is in her last year of classes. She has a scholarship to a prestigious university nearby, but only if she keeps up her high grades. She has very little appetite and has lost 5 kilograms. She feels hopeless and at times she believes that life is not worth living. She says that she would not do anything to end her life. She denies any alcohol or drug use. Jemila does not want to take any medication, due to fear of not being "normal."

Jemila left Afghanistan at the age of 9 years with her parents, two older brothers and two younger sisters. Her family lost their family home during the war, and she witnessed the deaths of two of her aunts and an older sister. Upon arrival in the USA, Jemila went to school for the first time and became fluent in English. She frequently accompanies other family members to the doctors to interpret.

Ngozi is a 38-year-old single man who presents to the health center in his South African village with abdominal pain. It is difficult to locate the pain in any specific part of the abdomen. The pain is associated with nausea, but he denies vomiting. He notes irregular bowel movements, but with no evidence of blood. Ngozi experiences intermittent pain, which is worsened by certain foods and alcohol. The current episode of pain has lasted approximately 3 months, although the patient notes that he experienced similar symptoms approximately 10 years ago. He says that he began drinking heavily at that time for 6 months after the death of his mother, but that he has cut down his drinking considerably since. He strongly denies being an "alcoholic."

INTRODUCTION

This chapter identifies the basic knowledge and skills that healthcare practitioners must have in order to adequately address common mental health concerns that are seen in primary care. We provide a general overview of mental illness, discuss the rationale for incorporating mental healthcare into primary care, and list strategies for the identification and treatment of common mental health issues by the multiple health practitioners involved in primary care. In many countries, not only physicians, but also nurses, nurse practitioners, and assistant doctors are the primary health practitioners for people with mental health problems. Community health workers and volunteers are also likely to be involved in their care. Every member of the healthcare team has a role to play in addressing mental health problems, based on their knowledge and skills, the time available, and the place of patient contact.

The cases described above are typical of patients who visit their primary healthcare practitioner with a combination of physical and emotional complaints. This combination has long been recognized worldwide, and can often frustrate healthcare practitioners who are used to identifying purely medical causes of patients' symptoms. The focus of this chapter will be to discuss the recognition and treatment of the types of mental illness represented by these cases, and of the other types of mental conditions that are most commonly seen by primary care practitioners.

Mental illnesses in different countries and cultures may present differently. However, their recognition and treatment by healthcare practitioners is vitally important. The World Health Organization (WHO) has identified primary care as the first point of contact with the formal system of care for patients with mental illness. The WHO charges primary care practitioners with four tasks:
1   identifying patients with common mental health disorders
2   managing stable patients with common mental health problems
3   referring patients with complicated illnesses
4   advocating for prevention activities in the community.[1]

We would add a fifth responsibility to this list, namely providing primary medical care for patients with severe persistent mental illness whose psychiatric care is provided by psychiatrists.

WHAT IS MENTAL ILLNESS?

Mental illness refers to a set of defined syndromes or clusters of symptoms involving an individual's emotional state, behavior, and physical well-being and functioning. Symptoms can range from nervousness and sadness to fatigue and loss of appetite, thoughts of death and hearing voices. The effect of the illness often impairs the individual's ability to carry out their normal social roles and functions at home, at school, and at work.

We recognize that mental illness is a Western construct that may not make sense to many people living in the developing world. Culture influences how mental health symptoms present and how they are understood and treated. For initial treatment, Western terms and explanatory models can stand beside the terms and constructs acceptable to a specific culture (*see* Chapter 6). Effective treatment can be achieved so long as the language and terms that are being used are in harmony with the patient's explanatory model (*see* Chapter 3). Increased public education and evidence of successful treatments are likely to result in greater acceptance of and less stigma around people with mental health disorders, which in turn increases the likelihood that they can be properly identified and treated.

WHY THE CONCERN ABOUT MENTAL ILLNESS IN PRIMARY CARE?

Mental illness causes significant morbidity and mortality worldwide.[2] The average life expectancy is 8.8 years less among people with serious mental illness compared with those without mental illness. For men with mental illness, the reduction in life expectancy is 14.4 years.[3] Mental illnesses are more prevalent in people with chronic and communicable diseases, and are associated with risk factors such as smoking, poor diet, obesity, hypertension, and treatment avoidance.[4] Suicide rates are elevated in many mental illnesses, leading to lost years of life and associated productivity. The WHO predicts that, by the year 2020, major depression will be second only to ischemic heart disease in contributing to loss of life years in terms of productivity and social functioning. The combination of mental illnesses, substance use disorders, and suicide has resulted in mortality and disability rates second only to those caused by infectious disease.[5]

Although the burden of mental illness is significant, the recognition and treatment of mental illness in primary care settings is poor, particularly in less developed countries.[6] Only 52% of low-income countries provide community-based mental healthcare, which includes primary healthcare. One in four countries do not provide even basic antidepressant medicines in primary care settings.[7] In a household survey of adults in 17 countries, only 11% (in China) to 28% (in Colombia) of individuals with severe anxiety, mood, and substance disorders in low- or middle-income countries had received any care in the previous year.[6]

The under-recognition of mental health issues exists despite the availability of effective screening tools and treatment strategies. Treatment of depression, alcohol dependence, and anxiety can improve physical and mental symptoms, reduce the use of ambulatory and hospital services, and help to improve functional outcomes.[8] Clearly, the role of primary healthcare practitioners is important in the recognition and treatment of mental illness, and in lightening the burden borne by patients, their families, and the community.

PRIMARY CARE MANAGEMENT OF COMMON MENTAL ILLNESSES

Different mental illnesses pose different challenges to healthcare practitioners. Mildly depressed individuals with somatic preoccupations and poor sleep have very different needs to individuals who abuse alcohol and request assistance with persistent anxiety. Successful treatment depends on many factors, beginning with the willingness of primary healthcare practitioners to acknowledge their important role in the recognition, diagnosis, and treatment of mental illness. Primary healthcare practitioners also refer appropriate patients to secondary care provided by specialist mental health practitioners and social supports within the community.

In many developing countries, practitioners must be aware of regional tropical diseases that may cause disturbances in mood or thinking. Malaria can cause depressive symptoms, mania, paranoia, and severe organic brain syndromes. Neurocysticercosis is a common cause of epilepsy in the developing world. It can also lead to depressive and psychotic symptoms. Sleeping sickness (human African trypanosomiasis) can lead to mood swings, mania, and depression.

This section briefly discusses the six mental illnesses that most commonly present in primary care settings around the world, as identified by the WHO. We review problems in their recognition and treatment, and briefly outline current practice standards in the treatment of these illnesses.[9]

Major depression

Once thought to be primarily a disease of the Western world, depression is now considered to be a worldwide phenomenon. According to the World Health Survey, the prevalence of depression is 2–15% among people with no other disease, and 9.3–23% among people with one or more chronic diseases.[10]

Although the features of depression are universal, the clinical presentation may vary widely depending on culture, language, and life circumstances (e.g. poverty and class status). The words and metaphors that patients use to suggest depression vary according to local custom and shared knowledge. Typical symptoms include sleep disturbances (most often insomnia with early-morning wakening), decreased energy, and poor appetite. Other symptoms may include lack of interest or pleasure in things, feelings of worthlessness or guilt, difficulties with concentration and memory, feelings of hopelessness and helplessness, psychomotor retardation or agitation, and thoughts of suicide.

The use of screening tools can be extremely helpful when multiple symptoms suggest one unifying diagnosis. Box 7.1 shows a depression assessment questionnaire that is commonly used in primary care.[11-13] Healthcare practitioners can use the initial two questions (asking about low mood/sadness, loss of interest or pleasure in doing things) for screening to determine whether further assessment is needed.

BOX 7.1 The Depression Checklist

The practitioner asks the patient whether, in the past 2 weeks, they have experienced any of the following:

Yes
I ☐ Low mood/sadness (hopeless or helpless)
II ☐ Loss of interest or pleasure

If the answer to any of the above is YES, continue below

Yes
1 ☐ Sleep disturbance (difficulty falling asleep, early-morning waking)
2 ☐ Appetite disturbance (appetite loss, increased appetite)
3 ☐ Concentration difficulties
4 ☐ Psychomotor retardation or agitation
5 ☐ Decreased libido
6 ☐ Loss of self-confidence or self-esteem
7 ☐ Thoughts of death or suicide
8 ☐ Feelings of guilt
9 ☐ Decreased energy and/or increased fatigue

Functioning and disablement
I During the last month have you been limited in one or more of the following activities for most of the time:
Self-care: bathing, dressing, eating ....☐
Family relationships: partner, children, relatives ....☐
Going to work or school...☐
Doing housework or household tasks...☐
Social activities, seeing friends..☐
Remembering things ....☐

II Because of these problems during the last month:
How many days were you unable to fully carry out your usual daily activities? ....
How many days did you spend in bed in order to rest? ....

Adapted from World Health Organization. *Mental Disorders in Primary Care.* p. 10; http://whqlibdoc.who.int/HQ/1998/WHO_MSA_MNHIEAC_98.1.pdf (accessed 8 January 2009).

Treatment would depend on the degree of dysfunction, how long the symptoms have been present, what the patient is willing to do, and the available treatment options. The recommended treatment for major depression is generally a combination of antidepressant medication, counseling, exercise, and/or support. In the developing world, professional counselors may not be available at all. In such settings, brief, evidence-based counseling can be provided by the primary healthcare team (*see* Chapter 8) or by others in the folk or popular sectors (*see* Chapters 4 and 6). Less severe depression may respond to counseling alone. Exercise has been shown to be a successful therapy for mild to moderate depression. More severe depression that involves functional impairment in major areas of life, such as work or school, requires the addition of antidepressant medication. Depressed patients who are deemed unsafe due to suicidal thoughts or risky behaviors may require hospitalization.

There is no evidence that any single class of antidepressants is superior to the others in terms of effectiveness or speed of onset. Treatment decisions are based on local availability of medicines, side-effect profiles, previous treatment response, potential drug interactions, and patient preference. Treatment guidelines suggest that single episodes of major depression require treatment with antidepressants for 6 to 12 months after remission of symptoms, as assessed by the primary care practitioner. Repeated episodes of depression and relapse rates are high in major depressive disorders, requiring ongoing treatment with an antidepressant for prevention of future episodes.

In the first case scenario described above, Jemila had several target symptoms that suggested a diagnosis of depression. She denied the symptoms of hyper-arousal and reliving of her war experiences, which are components of post-traumatic stress disorder (see below). Her primary care physician explained the diagnosis of depression and how it related to her symptoms. She stated that she had put these images behind her. He noted that her condition was both common and treatable, and that the basics of treatment included both medication and talking therapy, beginning with his own supportive listening to her concerns. When she had heard his explanation of the diagnosis of depression, Jemila agreed to a trial of an antidepressant medication.

Anxiety disorders

Prevalence rates for anxiety disorders around the world vary widely, from 2.2% to 28%, depending on the survey.[14] Only about 25% of individuals with anxiety disorders worldwide receive any kind of treatment.[15] The central feature of anxiety is an inability to regulate fear or worry. However, sleep difficulties and somatic complaints such as chest pain, palpitations, respiratory difficulty, and headache symptoms may be more common presenting symptoms in developing countries.

Panic and generalized anxiety disorders are the most common anxiety disorders with which patients present to healthcare practitioners. The central feature of a panic attack is the sudden onset of intense worry, with physiological reactions of racing heart, shortness of breath, tightness and sometimes pain in the chest, a tingling sensation in the extremities, sweating, and dizziness. A panic attack may be accompanied by intense fear of dying. Many people will go to their healthcare practitioner and report fears that they are having a heart attack. People with panic disorder have anticipatory anxiety about having a panic attack, and will begin to restrict their life by avoiding crowds or enclosed spaces, and sometimes they reach the point where they will not leave their home.

Generalized anxiety disorder is characterized by chronic, unrealistic, and excessive worrying. It is accompanied by sleep difficulties, feeling anxious or on edge, restlessness, irritability, fatigue, and catastrophic thinking (*see* Chapter 3).

Post-traumatic stress disorder (PTSD) is particularly common in countries experiencing war or natural disasters, but it can also occur in people who have experienced abuse or trauma (e.g. an automobile accident or medical procedure). Its central features are emotional numbness, an intense "startle" response (hyper-arousal), and an intrusive reliving of the traumatic event, often brought on by what are perceived to be associated "cues" in the person's environment. Sleep difficulties, anger or irritability, and fatigue are also common features. Alcohol and other substance abuse disorders are common in individuals with PTSD, who may try to use these substances to numb their emotional pain. Unfortunately, substance abuse only worsens the symptoms and decreases the patient's ability to manage their pain. As in Jemila's case, many refugees who leave their homes in war-torn countries do not want to discuss their recent trauma.

Box 7.2 illustrates an anxiety assessment tool that is commonly used in primary care.[11] The first two questions (about feeling tense or anxious and being worried about things) are the screening questions that determine whether further assessment is needed. Clearly defined treatment algorithms have been developed for primary care practitioners to diagnose the type of anxiety disorder and the accompanying depression and substance use disorders.[11]

BOX 7.2 The Anxiety Checklist

The practitioner asks the patient whether, in the last 2 weeks, they have experienced any of the following:

Yes
I ☐ Feeling tense or anxious
II ☐ Being very worried about things

If the answer to any of the above is YES, continue below
1 ☐ Symptoms of arousal and anxiety
2 ☐ Has experienced intense or sudden fear unexpectedly or for no apparent reason.
3 If yes, mark any of the relevant items below:
   Fear of dying .... ☐ Fear of losing control .... ☐
   Pounding heart .... ☐ Sweating .... ☐
   Trembling or shaking .... ☐ Chest pains or difficulty breathing .... ☐
   Feeling dizzy, lightheaded or faint .... ☐ Numbness or tingling sensations ..... ☐
   Feelings of unreality .... ☐ Nausea .... ☐
4 ☐ Experiences of fear/anxiety in specific situations. If yes, mark any of the relevant items below:
   Leaving familiar places .... ☐
   Traveling alone (e.g. by train, car, plane) .... ☐
   Crowds or enclosed spaces/public places .... ☐

5 ☐ Experiences of fear/anxiety in social situations. If yes, mark any of the relevant items below:

Speaking in front of others..☐
Social events...☐
Eating in front of others ....☐
Worrying a lot about what others think, or self-consciousness ....☐

Functioning and disablement

I During the last month have you been limited in one or more of the following activities most of the time:

Self-care: bathing, dressing, eating ....☐
Family relationships: partner, children, relatives ....☐
Going to work or school..☐
Doing housework or household tasks..☐
Social activities, seeing friends...☐
Remembering things ....☐

II Because of these problems during the last month:

How many days were you unable to fully carry out your usual
daily activities? ....

How many days did you spend in bed in order to rest? ....

Summing up:

Positive responses to I or II and negative responses to 2, 3, and 4: indicates
generalized anxiety.

Positive responses to 1 and 2: indicates **panic disorder**.

Positive responses to 1 and 3: indicates **agoraphobia**.

Positive responses to 1 and 4: indicates **social phobia**.

World Health Organization. *Mental Disorders in Primary Care*. p. 10; http://whqlibdoc.who.int/HQ/1998/WHO_MSA_MNHIEAC_98.1.pdf (accessed 8 January 2009).

Pharmacological interventions are the foundation of treatment for anxiety disorders, depending on patient dysfunction, distress, personal choice and availability of treatment options. Selective serotonin reuptake inhibitors (SSRIs) have been demonstrated to be effective in treating anxiety disorders. If SSRIs are unavailable, tricyclic antidepressants (TCAs) can be used. Benzodiazepines and sedatives can be helpful for short-term treatment or as brief adjuncts to treatment with SSRIs. Unfortunately, however, benzodiazepines carry a risk of dependence or abuse. Therefore care should be taken to offer other medications as first-line treatment. Benzodiazepines should not be prescribed for patients with a history of substance abuse, which frequently presents as a comorbid disorder in individuals with anxiety disorders. Although benzodiazepines may produce fairly rapid relief from symptoms of anxiety, the SSRIs and TCAs can provide greater long-term mood stability, as they become effective over a 4- to 6-week period. Primary care practitioners can effectively counsel patients, teaching them behavioral skills to combat the symptoms of anxiety, in order to lessen the burden of the disorder and help to prevent relapse.[14]

Counseling approaches include deep breathing, relaxation training, cognitive–behavioral therapy, and exposure therapy, where patients are very gradually introduced to increasingly anxiety-provoking situations, coupling this with the relaxation methods learned earlier (*see* Chapter 3). Zen or other meditation practices have long been used in Asian cultures, and are now recognized throughout the world as a way of minimizing symptoms of anxiety.

Somatoform disorders

Worldwide, 15% of patients in primary care settings report symptoms that have no physiological basis – symptoms that patients attribute to a physical illness for which they seek treatment.[15] These patients may suffer from a somatoform disorder, an illness that often coexists with depression, anxiety, or substance abuse disorders. Although standard diagnostic criteria may overly exclude many of these patients from a formal diagnosis of somatoform disorder, sometimes patients who use increased amounts of primary healthcare services may also undergo unnecessary and expensive medical evaluations and procedures.[16]

A reasonable and effective treatment approach includes the following:

1 screening for the presence of other mental illnesses, such as depression or PTSD
2 seeing the patient at regular intervals
3 excluding a medical basis for each complaint
4 clarifying treatment outcome expectations with the patient
5 anticipating and discussing with the patient any side-effects that might be expected from treatment.[17]

An understanding of the patient's symptoms does not always occur in a manner that allows for a consistent diagnosis. When considering a diagnosis of somatoform disorder, healthcare practitioners need to address the concerns of patients and educate them about their diagnosis. Chapter 3 provides a detailed review of interviewing and counseling strategies that healthcare practitioners can use with patients who have somatoform disorders.

Sleep problems

Sleep problems are common worldwide, with cross-national studies estimating that about one in four people identify themselves as not sleeping well.[18] The prevalence of insomnia that presents with daytime consequences of sleepiness, concentration difficulties, or difficulty performing daily tasks was markedly lower, estimated at approximately 10% of people worldwide.[18,19] Clinically significant sleep problems are characterized by four presenting symptoms, namely difficulty falling asleep, difficulty staying asleep, waking up too early in the morning, or waking up feeling unrefreshed. These symptoms are considered to be *transient* if they occur on four nights or less, *acute* if they occur on two or more nights per week for two weeks, and *chronic* if they occur on three or more nights per week for four or more weeks.[20] Symptoms are frequently more common in elderly patients, with some experts suggesting that they affect over 50% of all people aged 65 years or older.[21]

The causes of sleep disorders, including insomnia, include medical and psychiatric etiologies (*see* Table 7.1). The clinical history is the best tool for gathering information about patterns of sleep and differentiating between possible diagnoses.[22] Special attention must be given to inquiring about other medications, repetitive behavioral patterns that may condition sleep responses, and medical conditions that may be underlying causes of insomnia, especially respiratory, cardiovascular, and neurological disorders. The use of stimulants such as nicotine, caffeine, cocaine and amphetamines contributes to sleep disorder, as does the use of alcohol, and the sleep disturbances may well persist after the offending substance has been stopped. Patients with sleep disorders frequently present to their primary care physicians with comorbid medical and psychiatric conditions that complicate the diagnostic process. A biopsychosocial approach to the assessment of both dimensions is recommended.

TABLE 7.1 Causes of insomnia

Causes of insomnia		Medications that may cause insomnia	
Anxiety	Hyperthyroidism	Alcohol	Herbal remedies
Asthma	Itching	Amphetamines	Nicotine
COPD	Menopause	Antidepressants	Phenytoin
CHF	Obstructive sleep apnea	Cimetidine	Pseudoephedrine
Chronic infection	Pain	Chemotherapies	Steroids
Depression	Periodic limb movement	Decongestants	Theophyline
Fibromyalgia	Restless leg syndrome	Diuretics	
Gastroesophageal	Shift work		
reflux disease	Urinary incontinence		

COPD, chronic obstructive pulmonary disease; CHF, congestive heart failure.

Treatment for insomnia begins with education about sleep hygiene (*see* Box 7.3).[23] Pharmacological treatment approaches are effective, especially for acute insomnia, in preventing it from worsening into a chronic condition. The mainstays of medical management are the benzodiazepines, although some newer related agents have recently come onto the market.[24] In general, treatment with benzodiazepines should be limited to less than 2 weeks, just long enough to re-establish regular sleep patterns. Counseling and cognitive therapy techniques are also effective in improving sleep disorders (*see* Chapters 3 and 8).[25] Attention to the underlying disorders is essential, whether this a medical condition, an addiction, or a psychiatric disorder such as a mood or anxiety disorder.

BOX 7.3 Sleep hygiene recommendations

- Minimize the noise levels while you are trying to sleep.
- Sleep in a dark room.
- Avoid bedroom temperature extremes (too hot or too cold).
- Reduce your caffeine intake during the day.
- Reduce the amount of alcohol that you drink.
- Reduce the number of cigarettes that you smoke.
- Avoid eating or drinking immediately before going to sleep.
- Exercise regularly.
- Allow some time to relax before going to sleep.
- Avoid daytime naps.
- Get up at a regular time each morning.
- Go to bed at a regular time each night.
- Avoid lying in bed worrying about not sleeping.

World Health Organization. *Mental Disorders in Primary Care*; http://whqlibdoc.who.int/HQ/1998/WHO_MSA_MNHIEAC_98.1.pdf (accessed 8 January 2009).

Chronic unexplained tiredness and fatigue

Chronic tiredness is a condition that occurs worldwide. Patients commonly present noting that, despite getting enough rest, they are easily and constantly tired, especially compared with their previous levels of energy. The prevalence of the condition varies markedly, from approximately 2% to 15%.[26] A higher proportion of patients in high-income countries report having symptoms of fatigue when asked directly by practitioners, compared with patients in lower-income countries. Interestingly, however, patients in lower-income countries are more likely to present in primary care centers with fatigue as their chief complaint.[26]

A variety of triggers precipitate tiredness. Physical causes can be found in 30% of patients with chronic fatigue by obtaining a detailed history, completing a physical examination, and assessing basic laboratory analyses. Psychiatric diagnoses, including depression, anxiety, and dysthymia, are the source of tiredness in more than 50% of all primary care patients.[27] However, approximately 20% of patients who present with tiredness have no identifiable etiology. A very small number of these patients have chronic fatigue syndrome, diagnosed when the functionally disabling fatigue lasts for more than 6 months and is accompanied by at least four other associated symptoms, such as sore throat, unrefreshing sleep, and muscle pain, among others.[28] The remaining patients have either transient or prolonged fatigue, depending on whether their tiredness lasts for less than or more than one month.

Although there is considerable variation in the treatment of chronic unexplained tiredness and fatigue, the principles of management are similar and are especially conducive to care in primary care settings. These principles involve a biopsychosocial approach, and consist of the following:

1 offering multiple consultations over time in order to establish a therapeutic relationship and provide ongoing support
2 judicious ordering of laboratory tests if available
3 recommending lifestyle changes if appropriate
4 promoting behavioral strategies such as relaxation exercises (*see* Chapter 8) and exercise.[29]

Medications such as tricyclic antidepressants, selective serotonin reuptake inhibitors, or other atypical antidepressants may be effective in certain patients. They are worth trying, although individual responses vary, and there is no conclusive evidence to support their use.

Substance use disorders

Alcohol dependence is the most prevalent and best studied of the substance use disorders. Prevalence rates vary from country to country, with a lifetime prevalence rate of 13% and a 1-year prevalence rate of 4% in the USA, compared with rates of 0% in some Middle Eastern countries where drinking alcohol is a crime. The rates of alcohol dependence are lower in countries with extreme poverty, and rates have been shown to rise as poverty decreases.[30] Approximately 20% of adults who are seen in primary care offices have a substance use disorder.[31] People with substance use disorders commonly present to healthcare practitioners with symptoms of fatigue, poor sleep, anxiety, or gastrointestinal distress. It is important for all healthcare practitioners to understand that patients are often able to reduce their daily use of alcohol following outpatient treatment.

Recognition of a substance use disorder is difficult and relies on a high degree of suspicion and a thorough evaluation of the patient. Primary care practitioners are in an ideal position to screen, counsel (*see* Chapters 3 and 8) and, if necessary, medically assist with the patient's withdrawal from alcohol (or drugs). For screening, the standard CAGE questions are helpful in identifying patients with alcohol dependence, especially since they have tested as valid across cultures (*see* Box 7.4).[32]

BOX 7.4 The CAGE Questionnaire

* Have you ever felt you needed to **C**ut down on your drinking?
* Have people **A**nnoyed you by criticizing your drinking?
* Have you ever felt **G**uilty about drinking?
* Have you ever felt you needed a drink first thing in the morning (an Eye-opener) to steady your nerves or to get rid of a hangover?

Two "yes" responses indicate that the respondent should be investigated further about the possibility of alcohol abuse.

For medical management, benzodiazepines can be used for alcohol withdrawal and agonists/antagonists for opiate withdrawal. Disulfuram is useful for relapse prevention in patients with alcohol dependence.[33] Developing a trusting relationship over time with the patient and their family allows primary healthcare team members to intervene at times of acute use or when the individual is at risk of relapse, and can help the patient to cope with the long-term aftermath of the illness, including the medical, legal, financial, and social consequences.[34]

Community services such as Alcoholics Anonymous, detoxification programs, and rehabilitation programs are important in supporting sobriety. Healthcare practitioners can encourage patients and their families to seek these services from local volunteer networks, such as the Women's Union or the Farmers' Union in Vietnam. In those parts of the world where such resources do not exist, working towards developing local community support systems could be an important therapeutic step for healthcare practitioners to take.

In Ngozi's case, in the second of the above scenarios, when his practitioner asked the four CAGE questions, Ngozi admitted that he had thoughts about cutting down his alcohol intake, that he was annoyed by his family members' criticism of his drinking, and that he occasionally needed an eye-opener to feel normal. His CAGE score of three suggested that alcohol abuse was likely. Physical examination revealed no signs of end-stage liver disease, although liver function testing revealed a slight elevation of transaminases. When he was presented with this information in a non-judgmental fashion, Ngozi continued to deny that alcohol was a problem in his life. His practitioner reaffirmed that she was concerned about his health, and that whenever he might be interested in developing a treatment plan, she would be available for consultation.

SPECIAL MENTAL HEALTH ISSUES IN PRIMARY CARE

There are other areas in which mental health issues arise in primary care practice. The most identifiable of these areas is when patients with severe chronic mental illness, such as schizophrenia and bipolar disease, present to primary care clinicians for routine medical care. In these cases, an understanding of psychiatric medications and their possible influences on other medical conditions is essential, as is being aware that people with severe chronic mental illness have an unduly high burden of accompanying medical disease. The second most identifiable area, especially noticeable in children, is the psychological consequences of physical traumas that leave patients injured and disabled. In Jemila's case she had come to see the doctor 2 years earlier with two black eyes, after having been beaten by her 30-year-old brother for not attending to household chores. A community agency became involved to work with Jemila's family around conflict in their home. Half of the lifetime cases of mental disorders are set by the age of 14 years, and 75% are set by the age of 24 years.[35] Early intervention in patients with mental disorders can help to reduce the morbidity over a lifetime. The third most identifiable area is the psychological effects of patients with common chronic physical illnesses. Inevitably, primary healthcare practitioners will deal with each of these concerns.

It is prudent for them to develop a level of ease with patients with these conditions, in order to manage them as effectively as possible.

CONCLUSION

The conditions described above are the most common mental health problems with which patients present to primary care practitioners worldwide. The management of these conditions is well within the domain of primary care practice, especially in collaboration with other practitioners trained in mental health issues. As with all areas of medicine, clinicians need to be aware of their limitations and know when to consult and refer as appropriate in their situation and as determined by the resources available to them. Rather than rejecting mental health as a field that is somehow foreign to primary care, practitioners in these settings should see it as an essential part of the biopsychosocial approach that is advocated by primary care. The fact that Jemila and Ngozi presented to primary care practitioners was no accident. It was with these practitioners that they felt most comfortable sharing what can be, for a variety of reasons, frightening concerns. It is within the sphere of primary care, too, that they should in turn receive the kind of compassionate care and clinical competence that quality primary care practitioners can offer.

KEY RESOURCES

- **WHO Mental Disorders in Primary Care:** an educational package that includes screening, assessment, and counseling tools for six common mental health disorders; http://whqlibdoc.who.int/HQ/1998/WHO_MSA_MNHIEAC_98.1.pdf
- **WHO Guide to Neurological and Mental Health Disorders in Primary Care:** provides detailed information on assessment, diagnosis and treatment; www.whoguidemhpcuk.org
- **WHO Noncommunicable Disease and Mental Health eNewsletter:** provides information for international action on surveillance, prevention, and control of non-communicable diseases, mental health and substance abuse disorders, malnutrition, violence, injuries, and disabilities; www.who.int/nmh/NMH-News-February-09.pdf (February 2009 newsletter). To subscribe, email mailto:LISTSERV@who.int
- **Your Guide to Healthy Sleep:** a US National Institute of Health patient publication that provides simple information about sleep and tips for dealing with jet lag, shift work, and other factors that can impede sleep; www.nhlbi.nih.gov/health/public/sleep/healthy_sleep.pdf

REFERENCES

1 World Health Organization. *The World Health Report 2001. Mental health: new understanding, new hope*; www.who.int/whr2001/2001/main/en/chapter2/index.htm (accessed 2 July 2004).

2 Murray CJL, Lopez AD. Global mortality, disability and the contribution of risk factors: Global Burden of Disease Study. *Lancet*. 1997; **349**: 1436–42.

3 Dembling BP, Chen DT, Vachon L. Life expectancy and causes of death in a population treated for serious mental illness. *Psychiatr Serv*. 1999; **50**: 1036–42.

4 Prince M, Patel V, Saxena S, *et al*. No health without mental health. *Lancet*. 2007; **370**: 859–77.

5 Unutzer J, Patrick DL, Marmon T, *et al*. Depressive symptoms and mortality in a prospective study of 2558 older adults. *Am J Geriatr Psychiatry*. 2002; **10**: 521–30.

6 Wang PS, Aguilar-Gaxiola S, Alonso J, *et al*. Use of mental health services for anxiety, mood, and substance disorders in 17 countries in the WHO world mental health surveys. *Lancet*. 2007; **370**: 841–51.

7 Saxena S, Thornicroft G, Knapp M, *et al*. Resources for mental health: scarcity, inequity, and inefficiency. *Lancet*. 2007; **370**: 878–9.

8 Wang PS, Simon GE, Kessler RC. The economic burden of depression and the cost-effectiveness of treatment. *Int J Methods Psychiatr Res*. 2003; **12**: 22–33.

9 World Health Organization Collaborating Centre, Institute of Psychiatry. *WHO Guide to Mental and Neurological Health in Primary Care*; www.whoguidemhpcuk.org (accessed 8 January 2009).

10 Moussavi S, Chatterji S, Verdes E, *et al*. Depression, chronic diseases, and decrements in health: results from the World Health Survey. *Lancet*. 2007; **370**: 851–8.

11 Hymen S, Chisholm D, Kessler R, *et al*. Mental health disorders. In: Jamison DT, Breman JG, Measham AR, *et al*. (eds) *Disease Control Priorities in Developing Countries*. New York: Oxford University Press; 2006.

12 Hymen S, Chisholm D, Kessler R, *et al*. Mental health disorders. In: Lopez AD, Mathers CD, Ezzati M, *et al*. (eds) *2006 Global Burden of Disease and Risk Factors*. New York: Oxford University Press; 2006.

13 World Health Organization. *Mental Disorders in Primary Care*; http://whqlibdoc.who.int/HQ/1998/WHO_MSA_MNHIEAC_98.1.pdf (accessed 8 January 2009).

14 Price D, Beck A, Nimmer C, *et al*. The treatment of anxiety disorders in a primary care setting. *Psychiatr Q*. 2000; **7**: 31–45.

15 Gurege O, Siomon GE, Ustun TB, *et al*. Somatization in cross-cultural perspective: a World Health Organization study in primary care. *Am J Psychiatry*. 1997; **154**: 989–95.

16 Ormel J, Von Korff M, Uston TB, *et al*. Common mental disorders and disability across cultures: results from the WHO Collaborative Study on Psychological Problems in General Health Care. *JAMA*. 1994; **272**: 1741–8.

17 Servan-Schreiber D, Tabas G, Kolb NR. Somatizing patients. Part II. Practical management. *Am Fam Physician*. 2000; **61**: 1423–36.

18 Soldatos CR, Allaert FA, Ohta T, *et al*. How do individuals sleep around the world? Results from a single-day survey in ten countries. *Sleep Med*. 2005; **6**: 5–13.

19 Hajak G. Insomnia in primary care. *Sleep Med*. 2000; **23**(Suppl. 3): S54–63.

20 Rajput V, Bromley SM. Chronic insomnia: a practical review. *American Family Physician*. 1999; **60**(5): 1431–8.

21 Monane M. Insomnia in the elderly. *J Clin Psychiatry*. 1992; **53** (Suppl): 23–8.

22 Rosen G. Evaluation of the patient who has sleep complaints: a case-based method using the sleep process matrix. *Primary Care*. 2005; **32**: 319–28.

23 Neubauer DN. Insomnia. *Primary Care*. 2005; **32**: 375–88.

24 Wolkove N, Elkholy O, Baltzan M, *et al*. Sleep disorders commonly found in older people. *Can Med Assoc J*. 2007; **176**: 1299–304.

25 Sivertsen B, Omvik S, Pallesen S, *et al*. Cognitive behavioral therapy vs. zopiclone for treatment of chronic primary insomnia in older adults: a randomized controlled trial. *JAMA*. 2006; **296**: 2851–8.

26 Skapinakis P, Lewis G, Mavreas V. Cross-cultural differences in the epidemiology of unexplained fatigue syndromes in primary care. *Br J Psychiatry*. 2003; **182**: 205–9.

27 Ridsdale L, Evans A, Jerrett W, *et al*. Patients with fatigue in general practice: a prospective study. *BMJ*. 1993; **307**: 103–6.

28 Centers for Disease Control and Prevention. *CFS Toolkit for Health Care Professionals: diagnosing CFS*; www.cdc.gov/cfs/pdf/Diagnosing_CFS.pdf (accessed 9 January 2009).

29 Elliot H. Use of formal and informal care among people with prolonged fatigue: a review of the literature. *Br J Gen Pract*. 1999; **49**: 131–4.

30 Meyers MJ. Substance abuse and the primary health care practitioner: making the diagnosis. *Fam Med Recertification*. 1999; **21**: 56–76.

31 Ewing JA. Detecting alcoholism: the CAGE questionnaire. *JAMA*. 1984; **252**: 1905–7.

32 Fleming MF, Barry KL, Manwell LB, *et al*. Brief physician advice for problem alcohol drinkers: a randomized controlled trial in community-based primary care practices. *JAMA*. 1997; **277**: 1039–45.

33 Chick J, Gough K, Falkowski W, *et al*. Disulfiram treatment of alcoholism. *Br J Psychiatry*. 1992; **161**: 84–9.

34 Anton RF, O'Malley S, Ciraulo DA, *et al*. Combined pharmacotherapies and behavioral interventions for alcohol dependence. *J Clin Psychopharmacol*. 2006; **295**: 2003–17.

35 Kessler RC, Berglund P, Jin R, *et al*. Lifetime prevalence and age-of-onset distributions of DSM-IV disorders in the National Comorbidity Survey Replication. *Arch Gen Psychiatry*. 2005; **62**: 593–602.

CHAPTER 8

Counseling in primary care

Julie M Schirmer and Nguyen Duy Phong

CASE SCENARIO

Nikki is a 29-year-old woman who has been brought to see her primary care practitioner by her mother-in-law, because of her chronic tiredness and malaise. Over the past couple of years Nikki has slowly lost her ability to function. Her mother-in-law does all of the food shopping for the family. The fatigue started two years ago, after the death of her husband from "natural causes."

INTRODUCTION

This chapter describes an overall approach to patient care and several different counseling models for practitioners to use in primary healthcare settings to help patients like Nikki. Primary care practitioners need skills in counseling, given the high prevalence of patients with treatable mental health disorders, and the amount of disability that will result if these disorders are not recognized or treated. Despite their prevalence and their major contribution to disability, mental healthcare needs go largely unmet, according to the results of a recent household survey conducted in 17 low-, middle-, and high-income countries.[1]

Given the scarcity of mental health providers in many communities throughout the world, treatment of these problems must be shared by mental health providers and primary care practitioners. Primary care practitioners must have access to and competence in using counseling models that effectively address patients' problems in the time it takes to address other common health issues.

In the case scenario described above, Nikki is experiencing increasingly debilitating and prolonged fatigue, which is a relatively common complaint seen by primary care practitioners. Underlying causes of fatigue usually involve a combination of physical, psychological, behavioral, and social factors. Astute healthcare practitioners will continually assess these contributing factors, counsel patients, and negotiate plans to address the factors that may be contributing to the patient's fatigue. This includes treating underlying mental health disorders and counseling the patient about their reaction to stress and lifestyle factors that may be interfering with their health.

For approximately 25% of primary care patients, a good history and physical exam will lead to a correct diagnosis and successful treatment of medical and psychological symptoms, or behavioral problems that are contributing to the patient's symptoms. If Nikki had poor sleep hygiene, the practitioner would have instructed her to limit her use of caffeine and alcoholic beverages and to avoid taking naps during the day. If she had a good literacy level, handouts would be used.[2] Often, however, treatment is not that simple. Nikki could have an underlying medical disease or mental health disorder, such as anxiety, depression, or alcohol abuse.

COMMON FEARS

Many primary care physicians and other health practitioners hesitate to inquire about patients' emotional or family issues.[3] Reasons for this include practitioners believing that such information is not relevant to the patient's medical problems, or fearing that they will be overwhelmed by what the patient tells them, that it will take too much time, or that they don't have the necessary counseling skills or support to deal with more complicated cases.

In many parts of the world, counseling has seldom been modeled by primary care practitioners. Psychiatrists and other mental health providers may not regard assessment and counseling as part of the responsibility of primary care practitioners, and may be protective of their role in the treatment of mental health problems. Communication between mental health providers and primary care practitioners can be hampered by rigid rules of confidentiality pertaining to mental health conditions.

Hopefully the data about the prevalence of and disability caused by mental health disorders have already convinced readers that counseling in primary care is essential. The evidence-based counseling models described in this chapter provide an overall approach and counseling skills to begin applying to patient care. The case scenarios illustrate how these models can be applied. Chapter 10 will describe successful models and ways of thinking about addressing the larger systems issues.

PATIENT-CENTERED MODEL OF CARE

The patient-centered model of care provides an overall approach and framework for relating to patients, in order to understand their underlying problems and set priorities for treatment.[4] The model supports patients talking openly about intimate details of their lives, without feeling judged or criticized. This may be a very different approach from that in countries where medical practitioners' approach to care is often perceived by patients as stern, critical, and unnecessarily probing. The patient-centered model is collaborative – it assumes that the practitioner has medical expertise and that the patient has life expertise. It works best when there is a continuous ongoing relationship between clinician and patient. Using a patient-centered approach, clinicians:

1   **explore the disease and illness experience of the patient**, including possible

psychological, social, and spiritual contributions to symptoms and the patient's perception of the illness (*see* Chapters 2, 3, and 8). Some of this information may already be known to the practitioner prior to the visit, from previous visits, or from "local knowledge", particularly if the practitioner or other team members live in the same community as the patient

2 **attempt to understand the whole person,** including the patient's life history, family, work, and social contexts (*see* Chapters 5, 6, and 7)

3 **find common ground** with regard to the patient's' explanatory models (*see* Chapter 3) and their management of issues. Steps include prioritizing goals, assessing readiness to change, and treatment plans which include agreeing on clinician and patient responsibilities (*see* Chapter 4)

4 **incorporate prevention and health promotion activities,** such as providing education on health enhancement, risk reduction, and early detection of disease, and lessening the effects of the disease (*see* Chapter 4)

5 **strengthen the clinician–patient relationship** by showing empathy, sharing power, caring, healing, and building self-awareness (*see* Chapters 2 and 9)

6 **remain realistic** about the time required to address problems and about the resources available to patients, families, the community, and the healthcare team. The time and resources available will be different in every country and setting[4] (*see* Chapter 6).

The patient's *locus of control* is important to the practitioner–patient relationship, and may provide clues as to how directive the practitioner needs to be. Locus of control can be external or internal. People with an *external locus of control* perceive their fate to be determined by external influences, such as family elders, God, or past lives. They are more comfortable when an authority figure (such as a doctor or other healthcare practitioner) takes charge and tells them what to do. They may need convincing that their actions or thoughts can be changed to improve their health.

People with an *internal locus of control* perceive their fate to be determined by their own actions, and believe that they are in control of their life and destiny. These are people who may have migrated to urban areas, where they may have more educational opportunities, and may have seen the direct results of their labors. People with an internal locus of control cope best when they have the resources (information, power, and time) to make their own healthcare decisions.

In Nikki's case, the fatigue started when her husband died. In response to further inquiries about his death, she admitted that he had died from complications related to acquired immunodeficiency syndrome (AIDS). She and her husband's family had kept this secret from other family and friends. Nikki was grieving this loss and feared that she and her 7- and 9-year-old daughters might have the virus. She did not feel in control of herself or her future (external locus of control). She felt hopeless and helpless in the face of this unknown situation. Immediate testing revealed that she was human immunodeficiency virus (HIV) positive.

Ideally, Nikki's treatment plan would eventually include highly active antiretroviral (HAART) therapy, problem-solving about living with HIV/AIDS, family counseling about acceptance and testing of her daughters, grief work related to her husband's death, and cognitive–behavioral therapy for her depression. The practitioner would assist Nikki in taking control of her life. Multiple studies from around the world have shown an increase in depression and anxiety among people adjusting to HIV-positive status. The higher the number of HIV-related symptoms, the greater the likelihood of depression.[5] Depression can affect self-care, treatment adherence, and subsequent disease progression. Hence the call by international groups to include mental health interventions in HIV/AIDS initiatives that incorporate sound research to determine effective treatments.[6]

ELEMENTS OF EFFECTIVE COUNSELING

Some common elements are essential to good counseling and are relatively universal. Given the right tools, a primary care practitioner who has successfully seen patients and families through previous medical crises is equipped to be extremely therapeutic with very brief interventions. In busy office practices, physicians can screen and assess the extent of the problem, and then refer the patient to other staff members for counseling, as they may have more time for selected patients.

Projects in many developing countries have successfully taught counseling skills to primary care team members, who can include physicians, nurses, social workers, psychologists, lay helpers, and community members. Projects that integrate counseling into primary care are being conducted on multiple continents and have reported a decrease in patients' symptoms, decreased psychosocial distress, decreased long-term or recurring disease, decreased hospitalization rates, and increased identification of mental health disorders, compared with usual care[7,8] (*see* Chapter 10).

The common elements that patients experience in counseling include the following:

1 **a feeling of hope** that receiving help will ease the patient's feelings of helplessness and hopelessness
2 **a therapeutic relationship** with a practitioner who is caring and concerned, and who establishes an atmosphere of acceptance
3 **a new perspective** on their problem(s), including new insights and problem-solving options. The patient realizes that there can be reasonable solutions which they had not thought of before, when someone else hears of the situation
4 **corrective experiences** whereby practitioners coach patients to experiment, even giving them homework assignments to do between visits. Gaining new insights, and a process to act on those insights, can change the way in which patients think, behave, or relate to themselves, family, friends, and the world around them
5 **repeated opportunities to test reality,** with practitioners following up on the patient's progress or on the results of their homework assignments. Follow-up may occur over the course of several days in a mental health hospital, several

weeks in a counseling relationship, or even months or years in a primary care physician–patient–family relationship[9]

6 **a continual assessment of harm** by their practitioners, whether due to patients' inability to care for themselves, suicidal thoughts, or homicidal thoughts. It is not true that asking patients whether they have thoughts of harming themselves will put those thoughts into their minds. Exploring suicidal or homicidal thoughts allows both practitioners and patients to come up with plans to address patients' cries for help.[10]

CRISIS COUNSELING

Several crisis counseling models are effective for people who have experienced trauma or crisis. Crisis intervention principles can be applied individually or in groups for people who have experienced similar trauma.

In times of war or national disaster, psychological first aid is effective when it includes providing protection from harm, exploring solutions for basic needs of food and shelter, and developing social support. Protection from harm includes screening people for suicidal or homicidal thoughts (*see* Chapter 7), and for the inability to care for themselves due to emotional shock or physical disabilities.

Small-scale studies have shown that cognitive–behavioral therapy prevented post-traumatic stress disorder with persons living in post-earthquake Armenia and Turkey.[11,12] Trauma and grief counseling have been effective in helping children in post-conflict Bosnia to make improvements in weight gain and psychosocial functioning.[13]

Post-traumatic stress disorder (PTSD) occurs in people who have had traumatic experiences outside the realm of most individuals – for example, in war, national disaster, sexual abuse, or physical abuse. It can also occur in people who have felt physically threatened, including those who have experienced bullying, sexual assault, moving vehicle accidents, surgery, or prolonged treatment of diseases. "Secondary trauma" can also occur in healthcare personnel who deal with traumatized patients (*see* Chapter 9). It is best if PTSD can be prevented, as it has significant negative effects on functioning (*see* Chapter 7).

BRIEF SUPPORTIVE COUNSELING

In brief supportive counseling, practitioners explore the background and stresses affecting patients' problems, discuss the physical and emotional effects on them, problem-solve, and employ harm-reduction techniques. The BATHE model of brief counseling was specifically developed by and for family medicine practitioners. Either the total process, or components of it, can be used during office visits when emotionally charged information arises. The BATHE model moves patients to an emotionally stable place by the end of the office visit. Using this model, clinicians "bathe" the patient, being more or less directive, depending on how much time they have available and how talkative the patient is in telling their story.

TABLE 8.1 The BATHE counseling model

Background	Tell me what's going on.
Affect	How is that affecting you? How do you feel about that?
Trouble	What troubles you the most?
Handling	How are you handling this?
Empathy	That's got to be difficult.
Supports	What supports or resources are available to help you with this?

Adapted from Stuart MR, Lieberman JA III. *The Fifteen-Minute Hour: therapeutic talk in primary care.* Oxford: Radcliffe Publishing; 2008. Reproduced with the permission of the copyright holder.

A 1- or 2-minute exploration of the problem provides a lot of information about patients' stories and the stresses that are affecting their health (*background*). The question about how the stresses are *affecting* the patient or their family reveals information that can identify factors which are contributing to their problems, such as an underlying mental health disorder. Patients may provide information about themselves or other family members who may be at more risk. The question "*What troubles you the most?*" exposes patients' perceived threats or fears, of which practitioners may be unaware unless they ask.

> Nikki was enraged that her husband had been unfaithful, had infected her and her daughters, and had then died, leaving her to deal with the consequences of his poor choices. She felt hopeless and helpless, and believed that her life was not worth living anymore. Despite these negative thoughts, Nikki loved her children deeply and recognized that ending her life would not help her daughters to deal with their potential HIV-positive status.

The question about how the patient is *handling things* highlights their coping mechanisms and the degree to which the problem is affecting their functioning. Nikki was isolated, anxious, and socially phobic. She had few sources of support. She felt a great need to protect her daughters from the outside world. *Empathic* responses can be a summary of the patient's situation ("*This is what I heard*"), a statement of feelings ("*Many people in this situation would be enraged*"), or a reaction to hearing the story ("*This is so difficult*" or "*I care about you and your family*"). Although often spoken from the heart, "*I understand*" is an all too common practitioner response that can trigger intense anger in patients. Practitioners can never understand exactly what patients are experiencing unless they have been able to "walk in the patient's shoes."

Supports or resources may include factors intrinsic to patients, such as financial resources, cognitive intelligence, emotional intelligence, and past successes in coping with tough situations. Supports may also include factors extrinsic to patients, such as family (e.g. Nikki's mother-in-law, who provided her with physical and emotional support), the health system (medication, counseling, rehabilitation facilities, and hospitals), the community (friends, women's groups, veterans' groups, religious groups, and other support services), non-government agencies (often plentiful during times of national disaster), or government resources.

LEAST RESTRICTIVE ALTERNATIVES FOR CARE

The concept of least restrictive alternatives for treatment is an important factor in deciding the level of counseling and treatment for mental health conditions. The least restrictive alternative means that the choice of treatment matches the severity with which the condition is affecting the patient's ability to think and function. Levels of practitioner intervention include practitioners:

1 *giving permission* for the patient to tell their story
2 *sharing information* about their illness or condition
3 *offering suggestions*, including brief counseling, medications, or seeking assistance from family, friends, and the community
4 *making specialist referrals* for more intensive care, including referrals to counselors, psychiatrists, or community rehabilitation programs[9]
5 *hospitalizing patients* who are at risk of harming themselves or others.[10]

The greater the patient dysfunction, the higher the level of intervention needed. These steps can be initiated by primary care physicians, with team members supporting and sustaining this type of counseling and care.

Nurses, midwives, or community workers more typically reside in the community and know the stresses of patients and their families. They can encourage patients to discuss their concerns with their physicians, inform patients that stresses do affect their health and healthcare, and assure them that their family or personal issues will not be discussed outside the office visit. This concept of confidentiality, where stories are not repeated outside the healthcare setting, is essential to making patients feel safe enough to tell their stories.

Other primary team members can alert physicians about what is going on with the patient, and can provide counseling that may be too involved for the time that physicians have available to spend with patients. Nurses, community workers, and non-specialists can be trained to effectively identify and counsel patients with mental health diagnoses.[14,15] This is important in low- and moderate-income countries, where there are few professionally trained social workers, psychologists, or counselors.

After inquiring about (*permission*) and hearing Nikki's story, the practitioner understood that she was asking for help and was not going to harm herself. He educated her about HIV/AIDS and HAART therapy (*limited information*), and he provided information about depression, medication, side-effects, and what to do if her depression worsened (*specific suggestions*). He informed her that the testing of her children for HIV could be postponed for a few weeks until her depression was better managed. He instructed her about HAART therapy and accessing treatment (*specific referral*). He reassessed her suicidal thoughts, and expressed concern about her state of mind (*empathy*).

They developed a plan together as to how to approach the testing of her daughters for the virus. She agreed to take her medication for depression, to pursue HAART through the district hospital, and to return in two weeks' time to have her depression assessed and to decide on the best time to bring her daughters in for testing. Although she experienced some shock, Nikki now felt more in control of her life than she had felt for the past five years. She was hopeful that she and her family could handle whatever was in store for them.

SUPPORTING TREATMENT ADHERENCE

Many physicians, regardless of the country in which they practice, believe that patients will automatically follow their treatment recommendations because the physician is the medical expert. This is not necessarily the case, even with the best physician providing the best education about the disease and treatment. Patients may be embarrassed to admit that they do not understand the information they have been given, cannot read the instructions, or lack the money to pay for treatment. They may fear that they will be judged or, worse still, shouted at. However, when practitioners use motivational interviewing techniques, they create a non-judgmental, supportive atmosphere, where they can more effectively address their patients' barriers to care, and support their compliance with treatment. Chapter 4 provides practical suggestions as to how practitioners can develop a motivational interviewing practice.

PROBLEM-SOLVING THERAPY AND SELF-MANAGEMENT PLANS

Problem-solving therapy can be undertaken through individual or group counseling, with or without physicians,[16] or it can be integrated into the workflow of a primary care practice for such issues as cardiac disease, diabetes, arthritis, depression, obesity, and chronic pain.[17] Group medical visits incorporate abbreviated practitioner visits with group psycho-education, problem solving, and developing action plans to improve patients' self-management of their illnesses. Self-management plans require the practitioner to coach the patient in:

1 choosing a behavioral change that the patient, not the practitioner, wants and is willing to achieve
2 selecting targets that are behavioral and measurable. For example, "*I will reduce my dinner portions by a quarter, 5 nights a week*" is specific and measurable, whereas "*I want to lose weight*" is not
3 achieving a "confidence level" of 7 or more, on a scale of 1 to 10, where 1 is no confidence and 10 is absolute confidence that the targeted change can be instituted. If the confidence level is less than 7, the plan can be modified to increase the likelihood of success and boost the patient's confidence.[18]

The practitioner assesses the patient's self-management plan at subsequent visits. They then may develop a new plan or modify a past plan, based on the patient's experience.

Problem-solving therapy calls for practitioners to help patients in:
1 identifying barriers

2 brainstorming solutions, including past personal successes. In a group setting, brainstorming includes exploring what others have tried. Outside a group setting, patients can interview others about their successes between office visits
3 choosing one or two solutions
4 modifying the plan so as to obtain a confidence rating of 7 or more
5 accepting praise from the practitioner about the fortitude shown.

Supportive healthcare practitioners can help patients to choose one of the following options:
1 solving the problem by leaving or changing the situation
2 feeling better about the problem by regulating their emotional response (*see* cognitive therapy in Chapter 3)
3 tolerating the problem or their emotional response to the problem
4 remaining miserable, which obviously is the least healthy option.

COGNITIVE–BEHAVIORAL COUNSELING

Cognitive–behavioral counseling includes techniques described in the behavioral change section, which are well outlined in WHO materials (*see* Key Resources on page 108). Cognitive therapy is based on the premise that people cannot automatically change how they feel, but they can change their habits of thinking to improve how they feel. Counseling involves identifying and educating patients about their patterns of thinking that are detrimental to health, such as magnifying negative thoughts, minimizing positive thoughts, thinking in extreme "black and white" terms, or forecasting never-ending patterns of defeat.

The basic principle is to rework these "toxic thoughts" and replace them with healthier ones (*see* Chapter 3). Healthy thought patterns include seeing "shades of gray" in situations and choices, letting go of feelings about a bad event, believing in change, being aware of choices, feeling that life is manageable, viewing obstacles as challenges, seeing the goodness in people, and learning to trust people. The extent of a person's untreated depression will affect their ability to modify their negative thoughts. Medication may be needed for those who are so disabled by their depression or anxiety that they have too little energy to focus on or participate in treatment.

Behavioral therapy is based on the premise that one's behaviors can be "toxic" to one's health. Counseling involves developing conscious awareness of those behaviors and replacing them with other behaviors. It also involves persuading patients to do things differently – for example, getting out into the community or workplace if they have been shut up in the house all of the time. Exposure therapy teaches self-calming techniques, such as deep breathing or progressive relaxation, and then gradually introduces the patient to situations that are normally stressful for them. Behavior therapy is very effective for patients who have panic and anxiety disorders; the deep breathing techniques are ideal for such individuals. Shallow breathing is a key component of panic attacks, and trips off a series of physiological panic reactions such as heart palpitations, chest pain, light-headedness, sweating, and tingling in the extremities. Both cognitive and behavioral therapy involve patients practicing these new techniques on a routine or even daily basis. The more these new skills or habits are practiced, the sooner and more completely they will be incorporated into the patient's life.

CONCLUSION

An overall approach to patient care and evidence-based primary care counseling models are described, and can be instituted in a variety of ways in primary care settings. Crisis counseling, brief supportive counseling, problem-solving therapy, and cognitive–behavioral therapy are techniques that any team member can apply to patient situations where a mental health problem is indicated.

KEY RESOURCES

- Patel V. *Where There Is No Psychiatrist: a mental health care manual.* London: Gaskell; 2003.
- **World Federation for Mental Health:** This organization is dedicated to the prevention of mental and emotional disorders, the proper treatment and care of those with such disorders, and the promotion of mental health; www. wfmh.org
- **World Health Organization:** can provide treatment algorithms, patient handouts, and educational materials for practitioners and patients; www. who.org

REFERENCES

1 Wang PS, Aguilar-Gaxiola S, Alonso J, *et al.* Use of mental health services for anxiety, mood, and substance disorders in 17 countries in the WHO world mental health surveys. *Lancet.* 2007; **370**: 841–50.
2 World Health Organization, Division of Mental Health and Prevention of Substance Abuse. *Mental Disorders in Primary Care.* Geneva: World Health Organization; 1998.
3 World Health Organization. *Caring for Children and Adolescents with Mental Health Disorders: setting WHO directions*; www.who.int/mental_health/media/en/785.pdf (accessed 15 January 2009).
4 Stewart M, Brown JB, Weston WW, *et al. Patient-Centered Medicine: transforming the clinical model.* Thousands Oaks, CA: Sage Publications, Inc; 1995.
5 Collins PY, Holman AR, Freeman MC, *et al.* What is the relevance of mental health to HIV/AIDS care and treatment programs in developing countries? A systematic review. *AIDS.* 2006; **20**: 1571–82.
6 Freeman MC, Patel V, Collins P, *et al.* Integrating mental health in global initiative for HIV/AIDS. *Br J Psychiatry.* 2005; **187**: 1–3.
7 World Health Organization. *Best Practices – Mental Health Services: Primary Care*; www.who.int/mental_health/policy/country/BestPractices8_SEARO.pdf (accessed 3 April 2008).
8 World Health Organization. *Caring for Children and Adolescents with Mental Health Disorders: setting WHO directions*; www.who.int/mental_health/media/en/785.pdf (accessed 15 January 2009).

9 Stuart M, Lieberman JA. *The Fifteen-Minute Hour: applied psychotherapy for the primary care physician.* 2nd ed. Westport, CT: Praeger Publishers; 1993.

10 Stuart MR, Lieberman JA. *The Fifteen-Minute Hour: therapeutic talk in primary care.* Oxford: Radcliffe Publishing; 2008.

11 Goenjian AK, Karayan I, Pynoos RS, *et al.* Outcome of psychotherapy among early adolescents after trauma. *Am J Psychiatry.* 1997; **154:** 536–42.

12 Basoglu M, Salcioglu E, Livanou M, *et al.* Single-session behavioral treatment of earthquake-related post-traumatic stress disorder: a randomized waiting list controlled trial. *J Trauma Stress.* 2005; **18:** 1–11.

13 Layne CM, Pynoos RS, Saltzman WR. Trauma/grief-focused group psychotherapy: school-based post-war intervention with traumatized Bosnian adolescents. *Group Dynamics Theory Res Pract.* 2001; **5:** 277–90.

14 Ali BS, Rahbar M, Naeem S, *et al.* The effectiveness of counseling on anxiety and depression by minimally trained counselors. *Am J Psychother.* 2003; **57:** 324–6.

15 Chien WT, Chan SW, Thompson DR. Effects of a mutual support group for families of Chinese people with schizophrenia: 18-month follow-up. *Br J Psychiatry.* 2006; **189:** 41–9.

16 Bass J, Neugebauer R, Clougherty KF, *et al.* Group interpersonal psychotherapy for depression in rural Uganda: 6-month outcomes: randomized controlled trial. *Br J Psychiatry.* 2006; **188:** 567–73.

17 Jabar R, Braksmajer A, Trillling J. Group visits for chronic illness care: models, benefits and challenges. *Fam Pract Manag.* 2006; **13:** 37–40.

18 Lorig K, Halsted H, Sobel D, *et al. Living a Healthy Life with Chronic Conditions: self-management of heart disease, diabetes, arthritis, asthma, bronchitis, emphysema, and others.* 2nd ed. Boulder, CO: Bull Publishing Co; 2006.

CHAPTER 9

Practitioner well-being

Cathleen Morrow, Julie M Schirmer and Nguyen Van Son

CASE SCENARIO 1

Dr. Hjong Linh is a 30-year-old physician who was born and raised in South Vietnam and then emigrated to the USA with her husband, a medical researcher in Texas. The couple have a 5-year-old child, who was born while Linh was in medical school in Hanoi. After three years in the USA working on English language acquisition and meeting the language requirements, Linh successfully joined a family medicine training program in North Dakota, where she moved, without her family, to begin her training.

Linh works diligently but has difficulty with communication and gets frequent feedback from patients and supervising physicians that she is difficult to understand. She was placed on academic probation in the second year of her training due to poor scores on the in-training exam. Faculty evaluations highlight concerns about her ability to formulate assessments and plans independently. Linh faces potentially prolonged training due to these academic challenges. Her husband is stressed by his full-time research work and the care of their young child. Linh worries constantly about the fact that her son is growing up without her.

(As in previous chapters, Dr. Linh's name is written according to the Vietnamese tradition, with her family name listed first and given name listed last.)

CASE SCENARIO 2

Ms. Mercy Achebe is a 32-year-old nurse/midwife who works in a small health clinic attached to a five-bed hospital in a remote village in Kenya. Mercy will see anyone who lives within a day's walking distance. She is frequently called to the hospital to attend to mothers during delivery and to assist the one surgeon, who visits the hospital twice a month. When she arrives at work in the morning there are long lines of patients waiting to be seen, some having waited through the previous day and night. She is frequently interrupted with emergencies and triage concerns throughout her long day.

Recently there has been a cholera outbreak, and the death rate among adults has been rising. Many patients are malnourished and highly vulnerable to infectious disease outbreaks. There has been considerable concern about the spread of cholera to the hospital and health clinic. The recent rainy season was especially scant, raising fears about a poor harvest. Mercy is single and lives with her family. Although she provides support to her patients and many community members through her work, she herself has limited support from others. She is frequently contacted at home at night about health issues and questions from her community.

CASE SCENARIO 3

Dr. Carlos Flores is a 40-year-old obstetrician–gynecologist who works in Western Guatemala in a large urban public hospital during the day, and in his own private practice, focused on general primary care, in the evenings. Carlos is well known for his compassionate care, particularly of the complex obstetric cases that are frequently brought to him from remote mountain villages. Dedicated to teaching, he works tirelessly to introduce medical students to primary care principles. He advocates regularly at the legislative level for family medicine training to become integrated into the Guatemalan healthcare system. Dr. Flores is married to a dentist who also practices in the public hospital by day, and in their private practice by night. They have three children, aged 4, 7, and 10 years.

- What common themes connect these healthcare practitioners?
- What risks to their health and well-being do each of these healthcare practitioners face?
- Can anything be done to help or support any of these practitioners?
- How might culture influence this decision in each of these cases?
- Should we help our stressed colleagues only if they ask for our help?
- Is it "not our business" until and unless a crisis provokes interference?
- What circumstances might lead us to intervene in one of these situations?

INTRODUCTION

The medical profession has extraordinarily high expectations of its practitioners. Regardless of the country, the structure of the medical system, the prevailing cultural values, and the realities of local practice, healthcare practitioners live in a world of high demand. The values of selflessness, professionalism, continual devotion to the needs of others, and adaptation to often rapidly changing circumstances are the hallmarks of providing medical care in virtually all environments. Not only are there widespread cultural perceptions of the importance of such values, but also we, as practitioners, have the same expectations of one another. When we are judgmental, or even unforgiving, of practitioners who do not live up to our expectations, we perpetuate a system that demands continual personal sacrifice, self-improvement, and altruism.

The concepts of practitioner wellness, well-being, mental health, and overall health are ideas that have cultural origins and influences. However, all healthcare practitioners can recognize the fundamental dilemmas facing those who labor to provide care for others. The demands of their work often put healthcare practitioners in direct conflict with personal and family needs. While innumerable social, political, economic, environmental, and psychological forces work to create unique dilemmas and solutions in individual circumstances, certain fundamental principles are critical to the emotional and physical well-being of healthcare workers throughout the world.

This chapter explores the components of mental health and the particular factors that can contribute to mental health disorders, substance use disorders and "burnout" in healthcare practitioners. It calls upon colleagues, professional organizations, and medical systems to take measures to prevent, recognize, and provide appropriate support and treatment for practitioners who are experiencing impaired functioning.

WHAT IS MENTAL HEALTH?

The World Health Organization (WHO) incorporates mental health in its definition of health as "a state of well-being in which the individual realizes his or her own abilities, can cope with the normal stresses of life, can work productively and fruitfully, and is able to make a contribution to her or his own community."[1] The US Surgeon General's report defines mental health as "the state of successful performance of mental function, resulting in productive activities, fulfilling relationships with people, and the ability to adapt to change and to cope with adversity."[2]

Research indicates that mentally healthy adults in the USA, compared with others who are not as healthy, have fewer missed workdays, lower levels of health limitations, fewer chronic physical conditions, lower rates of healthcare use, and higher levels of psychosocial functioning.[3] This research measures mental health on the three scales of emotional well-being, psychological functioning, and social functioning.[4] It defines mental health as *flourishing* if one has high scores on at least one measure of emotional well-being and on more than six measures of psychological and social functioning (*see* Table 9.1). This model provides a general map for attaining mental health, with the caution that some of these dimensions, such as autonomy or environmental mastery, are culturally specific and would therefore require culturally appropriate modifications. What is normal in one culture is not necessarily normal in another.

TABLE 9.1 Dimensions that reflect mental health

Emotional well-being

Positive affect	Regularly cheerful, interested in life, happy, calm, peaceful, full of life.
Avowed quality of life	Mostly or highly satisfied with life overall.

Psychological functioning

Self-acceptance	Demonstrates positive attitudes toward self, acknowledges and likes most parts of self and personality.
Personal growth	Seeks challenges, has insight into own potential, feels a sense of continued development.
Purpose in life	Finds own life has direction and meaning.
Environmental mastery	Exercises ability to select, manage, and mold personal environment to meet needs.
Autonomy	Is guided by own, socially accepted, internal standards and values.
Positive relationships with others	Has, or can form, warm, trusting personal relationships.

Social functioning

Social acceptance	Holds positive attitudes towards, acknowledges, and is accepting of human differences.
Social actualization	Believes people, groups, and society have potential and can evolve or grow positively.
Social contribution	Sees own daily activities as useful to and valued by society and others.
Social coherence	Interested in society and social life and finds them meaningful and somewhat intelligible.
Social integration	Has a sense of belonging to, and of comfort and support from, a community.

Adapted from Keyes CLM. Mental illness and/or mental health? Investigating axioms of the complete state model of health. *J Consult Clin Psychol.* 2005; **73**: 543–8.

Mental health is a goal for practitioners who are working in any healthcare system. Most recognize how challenging this can be to achieve. The very nature of the work would seem to conspire against accomplishing this simple goal. Healthcare systems are extraordinarily stressed throughout the world. Patients are struck by illness at any and all hours, babies are born at unpredictable times, trauma is commonplace, and infectious disease can break out and become widespread in a matter of days. Healthcare practitioners have no control over any of this, and a sense of helplessness in the face of such uncertainty and unpredictability can be overwhelming.

THE EXTENT OF PRACTITIONER HEALTH AND WELL-BEING

There is little data on the mental health and well-being of physicians and other healthcare practitioners worldwide. Literature focusing on practitioner health tends to focus on alcoholism, substance abuse, depression, and suicide, and much of the available data on these is decades old. There are even fewer global data available about specific mental health diagnoses of healthcare practitioners. The following discussion relies heavily upon data from the USA and Western Europe, because these are the only data available. We acknowledge the considerable risk in extrapolating these data to other regions, particularly in the developing world. This is a genuine but unavoidable limitation. Similarly, the focus here is limited to data that relate specifically to physicians, as these are the only data available. In no way is this meant to exclude other healthcare workers for whom these issues are just as relevant. It is our hope that, at the very least, these data can be used as a springboard for discussion about health and wellness issues that are of critical importance to all practitioners.

The fundamentals of good health (i.e. healthy diet, regular exercise, adequate rest and sleep, sufficient recreation, social interaction, and meaningful involvement in one's family and community) are well known to all practitioners. Yet perhaps no occupational group is at such risk of failing to "practice what it preaches." Those physicians who are in good health or who try to improve their health are more likely to counsel and educate patients about health promotion and disease prevention.[5,6] The opposite is true for those physicians who are unhealthy.

Physician mortality is generally lower than that of the general population. However, physicians as a group tend to self-diagnose and self-prescribe, and are less likely than the general public to use formal health services.[7] Research indicates that female physicians, compared with their male counterparts, are more likely to report their health as being better than that of the general population, to have a higher rate of taking sick leave, and to utilize formal health services more frequently.[8] Rates of illness are similar between the genders, and physicians overall consult colleagues less often and self-treat more often than the general population. Child and adult psychiatrists are more likely to consult colleagues about general illness than others, and they are more likely to have laboratory investigations undertaken. This general tendency of physicians to avoid formal medical care, to self-diagnose and prescribe, and to work through their illness without the help of others is a fundamental risk factor for their well-being, particularly when issues of physical, emotional, or mental health are in question.

While research studies of physician health and impairment tend to focus mainly on mental health, substance abuse, and suicide, it must be noted that medical morbidity contributes enormously to work-related stress. Healthcare practitioners get diseases like any other members of the population, and chronic diseases have negative effects on their functioning at work. Many practitioners do not disclose illness, because the medical culture promotes the mistaken belief that disease is evidence of weakness. Therefore practitioners who admit that they are ill run the risk of demeaning themselves in the eyes of colleagues or patients and diminishing their worth as physicians. This factor contributes to a greater likelihood of self-diagnosis, self-prescribing, and poorer overall quality of care for physicians.[9]

TOBACCO USE

Physicians in the USA have led the way in reducing their use of tobacco products, with a nationwide rate now down to less than 4% of physicians, compared with tobacco use rates of roughly 20–25% in the general population.[10] Tobacco use among physicians is much higher in other parts of the world, particularly in parts of Asia, the Middle East, and eastern European countries, with rates ranging from 15% to 49%.[11] Studies support the contention that physicians who smoke tobacco are less likely to have the knowledge, skills, and attitudes to assist patients in tobacco cessation counseling.

Clearly, the significant and ongoing increase in tobacco use in the developing world has major worldwide health implications. Practitioners who stop smoking not only reduce multiple personal health risks of cardiovascular disease, lung disease, and loss of work productivity, but also model healthy behavioral change to their patients and communities (*see* Chapter 3).

BURNOUT

Burnout is a pathological syndrome that is well described and validated in the developed world. It is sometimes confused with depression, although it is distinct from it. Burnout is a syndrome of emotional and physician exhaustion and severe pessimism that results from prolonged exposure to stress. It may lead to diminished empathy and withdrawal, both personally and professionally. Compassion fatigue, a form of burnout, is a deep sense of exhaustion accompanied by acute emotional pain. The exhaustion affects the physical, emotional, spiritual, and social aspects of a person's life.[12]

> Mercy Achebe is at high risk of suffering from burnout or compassion fatigue. Her health system is strained for resources. She is required to do large amounts of paperwork, which she does late into most nights. She is lucky in that she has a supervisor at the district hospital who tries to contact her regularly and provide occasional relief for additional skills training. She has a well-established support network among her family and friends. At this point in time, Mercy appears to be functioning at a higher level than most of her peers, and seems to be balancing her responsibilities at work and at home. What would her supervisors need to look for in order to screen for burnout in their employees?

Burnout has three well-documented dimensions:
1 emotional exhaustion
2 depersonalization and cynicism
3 feelings of inefficacy and low personal achievement.[13]

Emotional exhaustion is caused by overwhelming work demands that drain an individual's energy. Depersonalization is characterized by an individual's detachment from their work, their family, and their own emotional experience. Inefficacy is characterized by feelings of lack of personal achievement, loss of control over one's life, and failure. The Maslach Burnout Inventory is a validated instrument that measures these three dimensions. It has been used extensively in studies involving US medical students, physicians-in-training, and practicing physicians.[14–16] Other burnout and compassion fatigue self-assessments are available on the Internet (*see* Key Resources on page 123).

In a study of more than 4000 medical students from seven medical schools across the USA, burnout was found to have affected 50% of students within the previous year, while suicidal thoughts had affected 11.6% of students within the same time frame.[16] A systematic review of 15 studies of burnout among physicians-in-training around the world showed equally high rates, which varied according to the study methodology and definitions.[14] A review that examined physicians' dissatisfaction with their careers found burnout to be a frequent complaint of practicing physicians. Female physicians were 60% more likely than male physicians to report burnout.[15] All of the studies associated burnout with increased risk of depression, suicidal thoughts, and suicide.

DEPRESSION

As described in Chapter 7, major depression is a leading cause of global disability. Healthcare practitioners are not exempt from depression, and may in fact be more likely to develop depression than the general population. Depending on the study, the rate of major depression in physicians ranges from 7% to 20% of the US population, with the lifetime prevalence being 13% for male physicians and 19.5% for female physicians.[9] Studies that have examined the impact of depression on the work of physicians have shown a decrease in work productivity, job satisfaction, and cognitive performance, probably secondary to reduced ability to concentrate. Surveyed physicians who acknowledge depression are two to three times more likely to self-prescribe and avoid seeking treatment than those without depression, due to privacy concerns and fear of adverse effects on their licensing and careers.[17]

Medical students are more prone to depression than their non-medical peers. Studies of physicians-in-training have found rates of depression in the range 20–25%.[18,19] Studies have indicated that the highest rates of depression among US students occur during the third and fourth clinical training years, that stigma is strongly associated with admitting to depression, and that students avoid seeking treatment due to fear of damaging their academic record.

There are no data on worldwide rates of depression among physicians or other healthcare practitioners, but worldwide prevalence rates of depression are in the range of 2–15% in community samples around the world, with evidence that the incidence is increasing in younger populations worldwide.[20–2] The WHO-supported Global Burden of Disease Study projects that the incidence of major depression is rising, and that it will become the second leading cause of disability worldwide by 2020, second only to ischemic heart disease.[23] This projection clearly has profound implications for healthcare practitioners worldwide, and for the skills and knowledge that they will need in order to provide adequate care for patients. Such a significant rise in prevalence raises considerable concerns about the health and well-being of all practitioners, as they have to cope not only with the burden of disease in their own patient populations, but also with the personal increased risk associated with an overburdened health system.

Dr. Linh suffered from depression. She was physically separated from her family, who she missed terribly. She was lonely, and she felt detached from her patients, her colleagues, and her studies. With encouragement from her advisor and program director, she sought professional help, which included medication and counseling. Her mood, energy level, and overall functioning began to improve, and she started to exercise. Her mother moved in with her so that her daughter could come and live with her, instead of living with her husband. She eventually completed her training and got a job in Texas, where she was reunited with her husband.

SUICIDAL IDEATION AND SUICIDE

It is well established that physicians are at higher risk of "successfully" completing suicide than the general population in the Western developed world. In the USA, 250 physicians die each year from suicide,[24,25] with male physicians having an up to 40% higher risk and female physicians having an up to 130% higher rate of suicide compared with the general population.[16]

A consensus panel addressing the prevalence of physician suicide concluded that the culture of medicine has given low priority to the mental health needs of its own. This reality has potentially serious negative repercussions on physicians' ability to acknowledge, identify, and treat mental health conditions in patients, colleagues, and learners. The panel recommended that changes are needed in institutional policies and professional attitudes to assist physicians in obtaining mental health treatment when it is indicated or desired.[26]

In general, suicide crosses most cultures. A recent cross-national study of 17 countries indicates that the highest indicator of suicide risk was depression in high-income countries and impulse control disorders in low- and middle-income countries.[27] Among the US general population, Caucasians have a much higher suicide rate than do Africans, Hispanics, and Asians. The only ethnic group in the USA with a suicide rate approaching that of Caucasians are Native Americans.[28]

The qualities that potentially place physicians at high risk of suicide include older age (over 45 years for women and over 50 years for men), experiencing significant relationship difficulties or serious losses, alcoholism, drug abuse, depression, anxiety, physical illness, change in work or financial status, excessive working hours, and access to lethal means of suicide.[9,27] Physicians' long working hours and access to medications that have the potential for lethality place them at high risk.

SUBSTANCE ABUSE

Substance abuse is a problem of increasing global concern. Since healthcare practitioners are a reflection of the population in which they live, substance abuse among them has important implications. Substance abuse can be broadly defined as the use of alcohol, narcotics, or any of a wide array of potentially consciousness-altering substances (legal and illegal) which impair a person's ability to function responsibly in their professional or personal life. Familiarity with and access to a wide range of substances is common in healthcare training and practice. A significant hallmark of substance abuse is denial, and it is here that the implications of substance abuse can become so devastating for healthcare practitioners and, potentially, for their patients.

The negative effects of alcohol abuse among healthcare practitioners are substantial. A study in 1988 found that among active physicians and residents in US training programs, 4% were alcoholic and 10% were "possibly alcoholic."[29] A survey of US physicians-in-practice found that doctors were less likely than their age- and gender-matched counterparts to have used tobacco, cocaine, heroin, or marijuana, but were more likely to have used alcohol, benzodiazepines, and minor opiates.[30]

Overall, rates of substance abuse problems among physicians are generally similar to rates among the general population, with a prevalence of 10–15%.[31] Physicians in the USA are more likely to receive more intensive and higher-quality treatment for alcohol and substance abuse than their counterparts, and are monitored more intensively for relapse, in view of the risks and responsibilities of their practice and work. The prevalence is highest in white and Native American males and considerably lower in Hispanics, Asians, and black Americans.

A study that examined risk factors for substance abuse across healthcare workers found that those most at risk were younger, were more likely to report moderate or heavy use of alcohol, expressed feelings of "pharmaceutical invincibility" (the belief that they were immune to the addictive potential of substances), and were more likely to have close friends who were abusing substances.[32]

Risk factors for substance abuse relapse were found to be significantly higher among physicians who had a family history of substance abuse, who had used a major opioid as their substance of abuse, or who had a coexisting psychiatric disorder such as depression or anxiety.[33] In general, physicians have higher rates of successful treatment and lower relapse rates than many other population groups, in part as a result of intensive monitoring and ties to licensing.

Dr. Flores was extremely overcommitted and passionate about changing the world. He had started to use drugs and alcohol to help him to function. His co-workers began to notice that he was having increasing difficulty in functioning. He would become easily frustrated and he made frequent mistakes, which his co-workers and staff initially "covered-up." They respected and cared about him very much, on account of all that he had done for their families and the community. Eventually the head of his department became involved, after Dr. Flores showed up for a delivery with slurred speech and the smell of alcohol on his breath. He was confronted and relieved of his duties. He eventually completed a substance abuse treatment program and agreed to stay drug and alcohol free.

Dr. Flores was not as lucky as Mercy Achebe or Dr. Linh. His alcohol and drug abuse had placed both his patients and himself at risk. It was not surprising to find out that he was separated from his wife and children, who had gone to live with his wife's parents. He and his wife had argued frequently over his drinking. His family eventually returned home and supported his continued abstinence from alcohol and drugs.

THE MEDICAL CULTURE

This review of major health issues affecting physicians highlights the need at all levels of training and practice to attend to the personal, physical, emotional, psychological, social, and spiritual well-being of all healthcare practitioners. A full consideration of health risks demands recognition of perhaps one of the most unspoken and unstudied hazards to physicians' health, namely the medical culture itself. Worldwide, the medical culture operates as a powerful force in the maintenance of the values of the medical system in which it functions.

The medical culture is a system which has, at its very core, a set of values, beliefs, attitudes, and rules, both written and unwritten, which are instilled through repetition over time into those admitted to its ranks. These cultural values have been born from longstanding practical realities about the nature of medical practice. This is work that carries extraordinarily high stakes and responsibilities involving life and death. It requires dedication, self-sacrifice, and innumerable hours of work to master.

Those setting out upon a career in medicine know that, from the very beginning, personal and family needs will often be secondary to the demands of the profession. This tacit understanding is implicit, given the years of work required to matriculate through the training process. Some conceptualize medical education as unnecessarily arduous, beset with unrealistic expectations of practitioners' ability to function in the absence of reasonable sleep.[34]

It is no wonder that medicine puts its own at risk. This is the reality of the work, given the complexity and enormity of training and practice. However, the failure to identify the risks to health and well-being, to support, educate, and promote the recognition of practitioners at risk, and to develop the skills to cope with these risks, is a significant weakness of most medical cultures. This failure calls out to all healthcare practitioners to pay careful attention to their own well-being and that of their colleagues.

PREVENTION

Primary healthcare practitioners know well the value and virtue of preventive medicine. On an individual level, much can be done to diminish the health risks of all people, assuming the availability of such basics as a safe living and working environment, clean water, access to adequate nutrition, and resources to support such fundamental infrastructure. Sadly, such "basics" are not available to a significant portion of the world's population, so the capacity for prevention varies widely across the globe.

Fundamental to adequate prevention for all healthcare practitioners are adequate, safe, and reasonable work demands, with some degree of control over work life, time for personal and family needs, sufficient rest, and recreational time for pursuits beyond one's work – in other words, many of the dimensions that comprise *flourishing* mental health, as described earlier by Keyes.[3] Early recognition of mounting stress, fatigue, isolation, loss of control over work, or diminished joy or satisfaction in work can contribute to swift identification of the problem and allow time for remedies to be sought. The value of a sympathetic peer cannot be overstated. A practitioner in complete isolation is a practitioner at considerable risk.

Resilience, or "the ability to recover from or adjust easily to misfortune or to change,"[35] is an important prevention concept. Resilience is a protective characteristic that helps healthcare practitioners to deal with the many demands of their job.[36] It involves commitment (a sense of purpose and passion in one's life), challenge (interpreting difficult situations not as threats, but as opportunities for change and growth), and control (the belief that one has the ability to improve one's life).[37] Table 9.2 lists multiple ways to build resilience.

TABLE 9.2 Ways to build resilience[38]

- Make connections with family, friends, and groups.
- Avoid viewing crises as insurmountable problems.
- Accept that change is part of living.
- Set realistic goals and move towards them.
- Take decisive action in adverse situations.
- Look for self-discovery opportunities.
- Nurture a positive view of yourself.
- Keep things in perspective – avoid blowing things out of proportion.
- Maintain an optimistic outlook.
- Take care of yourself physically, emotionally, and socially.
- Add ways of strengthening your resilience, such as recreation activities, meditation, and the arts.

Adapted from American Psychological Association. *The Road to Resilience*; www.apahelpcenter.org/featuredtopics/feature.php?id=6&ch=4 (accessed 25 January 2009).

RECOGNITION

Individual practitioners and trainees have a responsibility to pay close attention to their own health and well-being. Those caught up in their work, enduring long hours, fatigue, and multiple responsibilities might fail to see that their own behavior or emotional state is putting themselves, and potentially others, at risk. Although work performance and the practice of good medicine is clearly a goal, practitioners must also be concerned with their long-term personal health and happiness. Fatigue, irritability, impatience, unkindness, or inattention to others may be indicators of a stressed practitioner. Mistakes in chart notes, prescription errors, forgetfulness about appointments or meetings, failure to follow through on clinical studies or test results, or inappropriate anger directed at staff or colleagues may indicate a need for reassessment of working hours, personal goals, or work structure. Increased personal use of alcohol or medication, particularly for sleep or for help with getting work done, and failure to fulfill important personal or family responsibilities must be recognized as potential early warning signs of a practitioner in distress.

DENIAL

Stressed practitioners often respond to their stress, regardless of its etiology, by working harder. Denial may be used against the demands of personal, family, or work life stressors. This kind of coping strategy is often utilized and rewarded during medical training, and it can easily become an automatic response, given the powerful social and medical culture rewards for increased work. Denial is a powerful weapon in the hands of a stressed practitioner. It can be an excellent short-term coping mechanism, and it can sometimes even be essential to accomplishing a particular task. However, prolonged denial can lead to crisis when genuine work ability, work quality, or emotional or physical health decline. Friends and trusted colleagues can be of tremendous help by offering simple observations of a practitioner's behavior. As in each of the cases described at the beginning of this chapter, denial helps the doctor to deal with difficulties for a certain period of time, but the risk of harmful consequences becomes more and more evident over time.

CRISES

For some, recognition of early signs of fatigue, emotional exhaustion, dislike of one's work, or a particular personal or family problem will be ignored until an event or circumstance triggers a forced response. Crises originating from cumulative stress may not be entirely negative in their consequences. They may serve a useful purpose in allowing an individual to re-evaluate his or her work expectations. However, crises have the potential to become serious dilemmas, forcing significant change that can be painful not only to healthcare practitioners but also to their family and work environment.

When crises strike, healthcare practitioners are traditionally inclined to "work through" the events by spending more time on the job and away from their family and friends. Medical systems stressed by crises brought on by lack of practitioners, increased patient demands, natural disasters, or outbreaks of violence demand service, often at the expense of the practitioners' well-being. Such circumstances are often self-limiting, with the prospect of relief at a specified time in the future. However, many situations are ongoing and demand collegial or systemic intervention. Medical systems in developed countries support methods for obtaining time away from work in the form of bereavement days, family medical sick leave, or mental health leave. Buddy systems are essential for practitioners who are working under extreme conditions. As all physicians know well, failure to mark important life events, celebrate births, grieve deaths, respond to illness or injury, and be present for one's own family and community during important transitions increases their risk of diminished health and well-being.

Intervening in the lives of stressed colleagues poses complex dilemmas. When is it appropriate for a colleague to intervene in the personal or private life of another? In Western medical culture, there is a longstanding tendency to ignore the problems of troubled colleagues, thereby further increasing the risks to patients. The prevalent attitude has been that the behaviors of colleagues are "none of my business" until they become so bad that they can no longer be ignored. Happily, these traditions are gradually disappearing as medical cultures evolve towards better and earlier interventions such as systemic approaches to complaints, increased emphasis on patient safety, and communication training to reduce poor patient outcomes.

Recognizing the potential for harm, most would agree that we all share some responsibility for our colleagues. As potential distressed practitioners ourselves, most of us remember a time when a thoughtful intervention by a caring colleague had a positive impact on our personal or professional life. However, there are equally likely to have been times when we experienced concern for a colleague, yet chose not to intervene. The decision to address a colleague's error or patterns of mistakes is never easy. Fostering a workplace culture of openness, mutuality, care for one another, and supportiveness during difficulties may provide the best foundation for deciding whether an intervention is likely to help or hinder.

SYSTEMATIC SOLUTIONS

A recurrent theme in the medical literature concerned with stressors to physicians' health is the impact of long working hours and the resulting physical and emotional fatigue. Virtually every health risk for which physicians are at increased risk is made worse by fatigue. The quality of medical care given to patients by exhausted doctors is lower than normal. Several high-profile US cases of poor patient outcomes have led to legal solutions involving decreased working hours for physicians-in-training.

In 2003, the Accreditation Counsel on Graduate Medical Education (ACGME) regulations limited physicians-in-training to a maximum average working week of 80 hours. Very recent recommendations by the same body include further reductions in working hours. These working-hour restrictions have caused significant alarm within physician training programs in the USA, particularly in the surgical specialties.[39] The European Working Time Directive required that, by 2009, physicians-in-training should decrease their working hours from a current maximum average of 56 hours per week to 48 hours per week over a period of seven days, with a minimum rest period of 11 hours every 24 hours.[40] This legislation defined working hours as total time spent in the hospital, whether working or sleeping.

There is no doubt that regulation of working hours for physicians-in-training has a positive effect on their mental health and well-being. However, concern remains that the quality of medical training is diminished by working-hour restrictions. Although it is difficult to measure, there is no supporting literature to confirm that physicians-in-training, because of this legislation, have decreased their experience of burnout, improved their quality of life, or experienced a decrease in the quality of their training.

Clearly, adequate rest and sleep are critical for optimal functioning. However, working-hour restrictions are only a first step towards reforming a medical culture so that it embraces the overall health and well-being of its practitioners. Systems that foster positive, supportive environments and that address dilemmas facing practitioners in a non-threatening manner are equally important. Balint groups, practice inquiry groups, or other reflective-style support groups appropriate to a country's medical system provide safe havens for practitioners. Cultural practices that create social space and time every day for colleagues to come together to discuss cases, tell stories, and reflect on their work and personal lives are important. Shared daily noon meals can potentially prevent the emotional isolation that is experienced by so many stressed practitioners in developed countries.

Healthcare practitioners who have worked in developed and developing countries note the irony of the erosion of such shared times in medical systems of the "developed" world. The importance of maintaining such shared time in all healthcare systems cannot be overemphasized.

In times of war, natural disaster, or declining economies, systems of support in healthcare systems often fail. Yet the courage to engage, with care and consideration, with struggling colleagues is an increasingly important component of a multifaceted system designed to catch all practitioners before they fall.

CONCLUSION

A medical culture that acknowledges the human frailty of all its practitioners, that does not punish or ostracize individuals for admitting to fatigue, fear, mistakes, bad outcomes, emotional or physical exhaustion, depression, substance abuse, and beyond is worthy of our efforts to build. Creating such a medical culture should be the work of all of us. If we respond with genuine care and concern to all our colleagues, and equally to ourselves, we can create such a culture. No matter where in the world we work, certain aspects of our humanity are undeniable. We need one another, we are responsible for one another, and our work affords us the privilege and responsibility to attend to that truth every day in relation to our patients, our colleagues, and ourselves.

KEY RESOURCES

- The Burnout Self-Test: www.mindtools.com/stress/Brn/BurnoutSelfTest.htm
- The Compassion Fatigue Test: www.isu.edu/~bhstamm/tests/satfat.htm
- The Resiliency Quiz: www.resiliencyquiz.com

REFERENCES

1 World Health Organization. *Mental Health: strengthening mental health promotion*; www.who.int/mediacentre/factsheets/fs220/en (accessed 25 January 2009).

2 US Department of Health and Human Services. *Mental Health: a Report of the Surgeon General – executive summary.* Rockville, MD: US Department of Health and Human Services, Substance Abuse and Mental Health Services Administration, Center for Mental Health Services, National Institutes of Health, National Institute of Mental Health; www.surgeongeneral.gov/library/mentalhealth/summary.html (accessed 14 March 2009).

3 Keyes CLM. Promoting and protecting mental health as flourishing: a complementary strategy for improving national mental health. *Am Psychol.* 2007; **62**: 95–108.

4 Keyes CLM. Mental illness and/or mental health? Investigating axioms of the complete state model of health. *J Consult Clin Psychol.* 2005; **73**: 539–48.

5 Wells KB, Lewis CE, Leake B, *et al.* Do physicians preach what they practice? A study of physicians' health habits and counseling practices. *JAMA.* 1984; **252**: 2846–8.

6 Schwartz JS, Lewis CE, Clancy C, *et al.* Internists' practices in health promotion and disease prevention. *Ann Intern Med.* 1991; **114**: 46–53.

7 Forsythe M, Calnan M, Wall B. Doctors as patients: postal survey examining consultants' and general practitioners' adherence to guidelines. *BMJ.* 1999; **319**: 605–8.

8 Toyry S, Rasanen K, Kujala S, *et al.* Self-reported health, illness, and self-care among Finnish physicians: a national survey. *Arch Fam Med.* 2000; **9**: 1079–85.

9 Harrison J. Doctors' health and fitness to practice: the need for a bespoke model of assessment. *Occup Med.* 2008; **58**: 323–7.

10 Frank E, Biola H, Burnett CA. Mortality rates and causes among US physicians. *Am J Prev Med.* 2000; **10**: 155–9.

11 Kumra V, Markoff BA. Who's smoking now? The epidemiology of tobacco use in the United States and abroad. *Clin Chest Med.* 2000; **21**: 1–9.

12 Pfifferling JH, Gilley K. Overcoming compassion fatigue. *Fam Pract Manag.* 2000; **7**: 39–45.

13 Maslach C, Jackson S. The measurement of experienced burnout. *J Occup Behav.* 1981; **2**: 99–113.

14 Thomas NK. Resident burnout. *JAMA.* 2004; **292**: 2880–89.

15 Zuger A. Dissatisfaction with medical practice. *NEJM.* 2004; **350**: 69–75.

16 Dyrbye LN, Matthew TR, Massie S, *et al.* Burnout and suicidal ideation among US medical students. *Ann Intern Med.* 2008; **149**: 334–41.

17 Schwenk TL, Gorenflo DW, Leja L. A survey on the impact of being depressed on the professional status and mental health care of physicians. *J Clin Psychiatry.* 2008; **69**: 617–20.

18 Givens JL, Tija J. Depressed medical students' use of mental health services and barriers to use. *Acad Med.* 2002; **77**: 918–22.

19 Rosenthal JM, Okie S. White coat, mood indigo – depression in medical school. *NEJM.* 2005; **353**: 1085–8.

20 Weissman MM, Bland RC, Canino GJ, *et al.* Cross-national epidemiology of major depression and bipolar disorder. *JAMA.* 1996; **276**: 293–9.

21 Cross-National Collaborative Group. The changing rate of major depression: cross-national comparisons. *JAMA.* 1992; **268**: 3098–105.

22 Moussavi S, Chatterji S, Verdes E, *et al.* Depression, chronic diseases, and decrements in health: results from the World Health Survey. *Lancet.* 2007; **370**: 851–8.

23 Murray CJL, Lopez AD. Alternative projections of mortality and disability by cause 1990–2020: Global Burden of Disease Study. *Lancet.* 1997; **349**: 1498–504.

24 Lindeman S, Laara E, Hakko H, *et al.* A systematic review on gender-specific suicide mortality in medical doctors. *Br J Psychiatry.* 1996; **168**: 274–9.

25 Frank E, Dingle AD. Self-reported depression and suicide attempts among U.S. women physicians. *Am J Psychiatry.* 1999; **156**: 1887–94.

26 Center C, Davis M, Detre T, *et al.* Confronting depression and suicide in physicians. *JAMA.* 2003; **289:** 3161–6.

27 Nock MK, Borges G, Bromet EJ, *et al.* Cross-national prevalence and risk factors for suicidal ideation, plans, and attempts. *Br J Psychiatry.* 2008; **192:** 98–105.

28 National Institute of Mental Health. *Suicide in the U.S.: statistics and prevention*; www.nimh.nih.gov/health/publications/suicide-in-the-us-statistics-and-prevention.shtml (accessed 5 September 2008).

29 Siegel BJ, Fitzgerald F. A survey on the prevalence of alcoholism among the faculty and house staff of an academic teaching hospital. *West J Med.* 1988; **148:** 593–5.

30 Hughes PN, Brandenburg N, Baldwin DC. Prevalence of substance use among U.S. physicians. *JAMA.* 1991; **267:** 2333–9.

31 Gastfriend DR. Physician substance abuse and recovery. *JAMA.* 2005; **293:** 1513–15.

32 Kenna GA, Lewis DC. Risk factors for alcohol and other drug use by healthcare professionals. *Subst Abuse Treat Prev Policy.* 2008; **3:** 1747–59.

33 Domino KB, Hornbein TF, Nayak, *et al.* Risk factors for relapse in health care professionals with substance use disorders. *JAMA.* 2005; **293:** 1453–60.

34 Howard SK, Gaba DM, Rosekind MR, *et al.* The risks and implications of excessive daytime sleepiness in resident physicians. *Acad Med.* 2002; **77:** 1019–25.

35 Merriam Webster Dictionary Online; www.merriam-webster.com/dictionary/resilience (accessed 5 January 2009).

36 Kenyon T (ed.) *Fostering resilience in faculty and residents.* Annual Maine/New Hampshire Faculty Development Conference, 18 November 2008, Lewiston, ME.

37 Kobasa SD. Stressful life events, personality, and health: an inquiry into hardiness. *J Pers Soc Psychol.* 1979; **37:** 1–11.

38 American Psychological Association. *The Road to Resilience*; www.apahelpcenter.org/featuredtopics/feature.php?id=6&ch=4 (accessed 25 January 2009).

39 Gelfand DV, Podnos YD, Carmichael JC, *et al.* Effect of the 80-hour workweek on resident burnout. *Arch Surg.* 2004; **139:** 933–8.

40 British Medical Association. *European Working Time Directive: background*; www.bma.org.uk/employmentandcontracts/working_arrangements/hours/ewtdbkgrd.jsp (accessed 25 January 2009).

CHAPTER 10

Developing behavioral medicine in international settings

Julie M Schirmer, Alain J Montegut, Christina Holt, Ellen Fiore, Nguyen Thi Kim Chuc and Pham Huy Dung

CASE SCENARIO

Over a period of 15 years, a team of US family medicine educators have been consulting in five medical schools and six communities in Vietnam to develop family medicine in that country. Behavioral medicine and mental health have been strong curriculum components from the very beginning of the consultation. Gains have been made in training, yet trainees are sent to communities and health systems which are not set up to support behavioral and mental healthcare in their primary care settings. Work is currently being conducted to continue the development of systems, supervision, training, and support for primary care teams who can integrate behavioral health into their practice.

INTRODUCTION

This chapter uses the authors' work in Vietnam to demonstrate the principles and strategies to consider when integrating mental and behavioral healthcare into primary care systems, where psychiatrists and other behavioral health "experts" are scarce. Later on in the chapter, we describe projects that train community health workers and nurses at the village and district levels of care to support primary care practitioners to assess and treat their patients' mental health needs.

The Vietnam project began with the introduction of behavioral medicine into the curriculum of family medicine training programs, and then expanded to include the training of other health and social service practitioners in Vietnam. There is a physician bias to our discussion, because the primary focus of our work has been with physician training systems. We recognize that, in many countries, physicians are not the primary healthcare practitioners at the community level. For example, in Zanzibar, the primary healthcare practitioners are nurses. In Tanzania, the primary healthcare practitioners are first-aid volunteers, the second level of care is provided in dispensaries, and the third level of care is provided by nurses and medical assistants. In Pakistan, the primary healthcare practitioners are health workers who have had only brief training, and the second level of care is provided by primary care doctors.[1]

Recognition of the need to integrate mental and behavioral healthcare in primary care settings is growing, as more and more countries make the epidemiological transition from infectious disease to more chronic ailments. The main benefits of this transition are an increase in life expectancy and general improvements in overall physical health. The main challenge is an accompanying increase in mental health disorders and behavioral-related disorders. The first reason for this epidemiological shift is changing demographics, particularly in the age groups at high risk for developing mental health disorders.[2,3] The second reason is the increasing rate of depression in countries as diverse as the USA, Taiwan, Lebanon, and Western Europe.[4]

Many inspiring pilot projects have demonstrated how to successfully integrate mental and behavioral health into primary healthcare. Projects in Africa, South America, and the Middle East have incorporated mental healthcare into primary care, with supervision and support from district healthcare sites and community mental health clinics. Where community mental health clinics are not available, district health centers become the referral centers for multiple community health stations. Yet district health centers are mostly located in urban areas. Shanghai, in China, integrates mental health services into primary care facilities at the district level of care. Services include medical monitoring, home visits, and "guardianship networks" of trained volunteers who supervise patients, provide family support, and help patients to maintain treatment schedules. These premier models are very effective. However, they are not widely duplicated throughout the countries.[5]

National legislation on providing mental healthcare at the community level has been passed in several countries, but legislation is no guarantee that it will happen nation-wide, since funding and systems development may be limited. Pakistan recently passed national legislation to integrate mental healthcare into primary healthcare.[6] Their model provides mental health training for primary care physicians and health workers, along with consultation by junior psychiatrists, and identifies priority groups for attention, treatment, and monitoring via a national health management information system.[5] The model works in urban areas, but adoption is a long way off in many rural areas of the country, particularly in areas where conflict is rife and civil structures are fractured.

In most developing countries there is a high degree of stigma attached to mental health disorders. Many such disorders are not presented to medical practitioners and therefore go unrecognized. Many medical practitioners do not want to address mental health issues, often due to lack of training and support. Depression and anxiety disorders often present as fatigue with multiple somatic complaints. Practitioners need the knowledge and skills to recognize the physical manifestations of mental health disorders and to treat the underlying disorders that cause the complaints.

BACKGROUND TO THE VIETNAM PROJECT

Our project began in the early 1990s as a partnership between the Institute of Health Strategy and Policy, which is a department of the Ministry of Health in Vietnam, and the Division of International Health Improvement of Maine Medical Center (DIHI) in Portland, Maine. The project goal was to assess the need for, and then develop, family medicine training programs in five medical schools in Vietnam. The goal has expanded to include training of nurses, social workers, and other members of the healthcare team. The project has included behavioral medicine consultations, curriculum development, multiple needs assessments, and on-site intensive training courses.[7-9] So far the team has consulted on behavioral medicine curriculum development to five family medicine postgraduate training programs, to representative medical faculty from six of the eight medical schools in Vietnam, to several schools of social work in Hanoi, and to provincial health administrators in Khanh Hoa Province.

Early behavioral medicine input to the project exposed family medicine faculty and key leaders in the Vietnam Ministry of Health (MOH) and Ministry of Education (MOE) to Western-based family medicine training models that integrate behavioral medicine into their curriculum. This work has eventually involved faculty from schools of medicine, social work, nursing, and public health, as well as healthcare administrators, managers, and staff.

Many factors specific to Vietnam have influenced and promoted the advances made to incorporate mental health and behavioral medicine principles and practices into primary care training. Since the beginning of the project, Vietnam's national economy has risen from an extreme poverty level to a moderate poverty level. The World Bank distinguishes between three national poverty levels using income as an indicator. Extreme poverty is defined as having more than 25% of the population earning less than US$ 1.25 per day. Moderate poverty is defined as having more than 25% earning between US$ 1.25 and US$ 2.00 per day. Relative poverty is found in high-income countries, where household income is below a certain percentage (e.g. 50%) of the average national income.

According to the World Bank, Vietnam is still classified as a low-income country, yet over the past 10 years its economy has grown at an annual rate of 8–20%, allowing increased monies to be directed towards health and mental healthcare.[10,11] Vietnam's reliance on centralized planning and centralized financing of policies has facilitated the implementation of health policies related to this project. Because of these policies, there have been increased opportunities to train in-country behavioral medicine experts through the project and through the 26 or more new schools of social work. These "behavioralists" will transform and teach behavioral medicine principles to physicians and healthcare team members in a way that is in harmony with the country's culture. The behavioralists can provide specialized mental healthcare for patients, identify community mental health needs, and educate communities about how communal health centers can meet these needs. At the same time, jobs will need to be created, reasonable pay scales determined, and financing for behavioral services addressed.

In Vietnam, as in other countries, untreated mental illness contributes to a cycle of poverty. Local Women's Unions, Youth Organizations, and Farmers Unions provide financial and emotional support to families in need, but they cannot treat the illnesses that contribute to this cycle. During the past 10 years, several laws have been passed to provide financial support and health insurance for the poor, for government workers, and for those who work in private companies that employ 10 or more people per year.[12] Yet many individuals are unaware that they are insured,[12] and medical institutions and practitioners have been slow to accept payment of health insurance.[13] Even with insurance, Vietnam has no systematic way of meeting the outpatient needs of people with mental or behavior-induced disorders. There are some pilot projects operating in areas with high concentrations of special populations, such as intravenous drug users and people living with HIV/AIDS.[14]

These challenges are similar to those confronted by the introduction of any innovation into a system of healthcare training. Yet the complexity increases when the healthcare system in which the innovation is implemented is different from one's own, when the economic resources are limited, and when trauma pervades the region. It is typical in low-income countries to find healthcare systems that are oriented towards urgent or emergent healthcare needs, where the structure and available time for practitioners to see patients is very brief, and where there is minimal training in the principles and practice of behavioral medicine.

In most of the developing world, primary care visits are similar to acute care visits in the USA, being typically 3 to 5 minutes long, with the focus being on only one problem. Many developing countries are facing an epidemiological shift away from infectious disease and towards chronic disease care. Despite this shift, medical practitioners have been slow to modify their systems to prevent, treat, and manage chronic health conditions. Furthermore, patients do not usually expect assessment and care in this arena, and may consider it intrusive if practitioners proceed in such a manner. Adequate consultation from psychiatrists is often lacking.

Many patients are hesitant to share emotional issues with healthcare practitioners. Stigma surrounding mental illness is high, and the nomenclature for mental health problems differs from the Western mental health model. Many mental health problems tend to present to primary healthcare practitioners as multiple physical complaints, with fatigue as the overriding symptom[15,16] (*see* Chapters 3 and 7). Physical complaints are more acceptable than psychological ones for missed work, decreased functioning, and treatment. Patients with severe mental health problems often consult witch doctors or fortune tellers before seeking help from the medical or mental health systems[17] (*see* Chapter 6).

THEORETICAL CONSIDERATIONS

We shall describe four institutional domains or "worlds" to organize our thoughts about establishing behavioral medicine in Vietnam or in any developing country. The domains are patterned after CJ Peek's "three-world model", which describes the areas to consider when integrating mental health into healthcare. Peek and colleagues recommend that every action designed to produce a change in an organization must satisfy the demands of the clinical, operational, and financial worlds.[18] We include teaching in the clinical domain and public policy in the financial domain, while we highlight culture as a separate domain. The cultural domain focuses on how medical care is delivered, perceived, and accessed by patients (i.e. the community culture) and by medical practitioners (i.e. the medical culture). Including a separate cultural domain provides the opportunity to reflect on the challenges of integrating a behavioral medicine curriculum into settings that are different from one's own. We shall first describe these worlds as they apply to our work in Vietnam. We shall then apply them to what we have learned from our family medicine colleagues who have worked in developing countries in other parts

TABLE 10.1 Behavioral medicine training and implementation strategies in Vietnam, categorized by domain

Clinical/teaching domain

1999–2007	Consultant presentation to Vietnam medical training programs and institutions on behavioral medicine content and teaching methods
1999–2007	Site visits by Vietnamese faculty to US behavioral medicine faculty
2000–2001	Curriculum development by local faculty
2003–2004	Needs assessments of potential behavioral medicine faculty in Vietnam
2006–2007	Assessment of behavioral medicine content priorities of in-country practitioners
2006–2007	Telephone survey of family medicine physician consultants regarding behavioral medicine content and processes in other developing countries
2007	Behavioral Medicine Certificate program provided to family medicine, public health, social work, nursing, and pharmacy faculty from Hanoi, Thai Nguyen, and Hai Phong,Vietnam
2007–2008	Writing team identified for book project

Financial/policy domain

1999–2007	Meetings with Ministry of Health, Ministry of Education, and medical school deans
2004–2008	Exploration of funding for specific behavioral medicine projects
2007–2008	Meetings and training to include medical administrators and managers

Operational domain

1999–2008	Meetings with medical school deans and faculty of departments of family medicine, psychiatry, psychology, sociology, and social work
1999–2007	Site visits to Hanoi, Thai Nguyen, Ho Chi Minh City, Can Tho, Hué, and Danang family medicine training sites, medical schools, communal health centers, and general and specialty hospitals
2005–2006	Review and input given on proposed national curriculum for social work training
2004–2006	Memos of Agreement signed with Thang Long University and a consortium of five universities in Hanoi to support curriculum development for Master's and Bachelor's level social work training

Cultural/community domain

1998–1999	Literature review of history and culture
1998–2008	Meetings with cultural brokers in the USA and Vietnam
2006–2008	Meetings with community service practitioners and non-government organizations

of the world. Table 10.1 categorizes aspects of our work in Vietnam according to the four health system domains.

Clinical/teaching domain

The primary foci of this project have been curriculum development, faculty training, and the appropriate placement of mental health and behavioral health issues within the primary care context. Through ongoing exposure, understanding of these elements has passed on to key leaders in the MOH and MOE, allowing the Vietnamese needs and culturally appropriate aspects of service delivery and care to be fully addressed.

Workforce development was evaluated with a 2-year needs assessment of potential behavioral medicine faculty.[8] At the time, there were no training programs that prepared behavioral medicine specialists. The few Master's-level-trained social workers or psychologists were trained in other countries and employed by non-government organizations (NGOs). The results of the needs assessment led us to become involved in the development of social work training programs at Thang Long University and Hanoi National University. A work plan has been produced that includes broadening our involvement in the development of ancillary mental health workers to work within the context of primary care.

A survey of family medicine department directors and associated faculty allowed us to see how they prioritized seven behavioral medicine content areas described in Feldman and Christensen's book *Behavioral Medicine in Primary Care: a Practical Guide*.[19] The survey results have helped to inform curriculum priorities, advising future training of family medicine and behavioral medicine teachers and clinicians. Most respondents listed behavioral change (*see* Chapter 4) as first and mental health (*see* Chapter 7) as last in rank order of curriculum importance. The other topics, listed from most to least important, were social/cultural issues (*see* Chapter 6), family community influence on health (*see* Chapter 5), physician well-being (*see* Chapter 9), psychosocial treatments (*see* Chapter 8), and the mind–body interaction (*see* Chapter 2).

Discussions with healthcare administrators in Vietnam have made it clear that many primary care physicians do not see their role as detecting and treating mental health problems. In the USA, family medicine training programs have accepted the role of physicians in the identification and treatment of mental health problems. Yet it is only recently that US training programs have embraced behavioral change as a strong role for family physicians, which is different from the Vietnamese priorities.

Financial and policy domain

In Vietnam, new educational efforts follow only after a need has been determined and a national policy directive has been issued to support the development of new curriculum priorities and care structures. In 2001, the MOH approved family medicine as a new first-degree specialty that should be provided at the communal level of healthcare. A first-degree specialty has a unique body of knowledge and skills that requires training beyond medical school. Before this, those who practiced in communal health centers were either assistant physicians with 2 years of training after high school, or medical school graduates without specialty training. After the MOH declaration, training programs were developed to support this planned level of care. The proportion of first-degree specialty physicians in communal health sites increased from 4% to 40% in just 5 years (2001–2006). Routine progress reports and testimony on systems outcomes are provided to the MOE and the MOH as part of our project.

Similar financial and policy changes are taking place to integrate mental health and behavioral health into the primary care level of education and service. In 2007, the newly appointed Minister of Health set a 5-year goal to bring mental health services to the communal and district levels of healthcare. The new minister, along with international colleagues, recognized that the concentration of mental health resources in psychotropic medications and psychiatric hospital beds did not meet the mental health needs of the Vietnamese people.[1]

Community health workers are currently attached to each communal health center, providing the bridge between the community and the communal health center. Community health workers receive minimal on-the-job training. They are often either paid very little (earning approximately 4% of a physician's income) or they are volunteers. In 2005 and 2006, the MOE approved a Bachelor's-level and Master's-level social work curriculum, and gave permission for 26 new schools to develop training programs in social work, a discipline that had been disbanded in the mid-1970s. The behavioral consulting team had the opportunity to provide input to the national curriculum prior to its final approval. These social workers will have upgraded skills to take on the position of the community health workers. Payment and salary scales are currently being studied for presentation to the appropriate ministries for official approval.

Operational domain

Administering a coordinated, educational, and clinical service program that connects mental and physical health concerns at the communal health center (CHC) level requires that practitioners learn new skills in operations. The CHCs have often been run as urgent care centers. Administrative and operational changes are necessary to incorporate mental and behavioral health assessment and treatment into primary healthcare. Supervision and support are needed from the psychiatric teams working in the district and provincial health centers. Collaboration with formal and voluntary community groups is necessary, whenever available. Referral networks must be established to identify and refer cases. Relationships need to be developed with NGOs, community support systems, and community mental health and substance abuse centers, where available. Psychotropic medications need to be in ready supply. Knowing how and when to address mental health and behavioral health problems, and developing links to community groups to support patient well-being, will be major steps forward in the services provided at CHCs.

Our Vietnamese co-authors continually bring new resources to bear on the development of programs that incorporate behavioral medicine into primary healthcare. At the beginning of the project, Pham Huy Dung, MD, PhD and Nguyen Thi Kim Chuc, PhD were top administrators in the research institute associated with the MOH. They are now key administrators, teachers, and researchers in schools of medicine, social work, and psychology in Hanoi, and are influential with national officials and professional networks in advising on legislation with regard to training, salary indices, and program implementation. Memoranda of Understanding have been signed, and funding has been obtained for consultants to begin to support the newly created schools of social work in Vietnam.

Cultural domain

Culture plays a significant role in any patient, systems, or community encounter, even within one's own community. Yet one has no choice but to focus on the cultural domain when consulting, teaching, or providing care in countries other than one's own. In Vietnam, much work needs to be done to shift primary healthcare practitioners' range of competency and care from an acute, biomedical focus to a biopsychosocial focus, where mental health and behavioral health issues can be addressed. As stated above, supervision and support will help to move along this cultural transition in which primary care practitioners begin to see mental health and behavioral healthcare as their responsibility. Training all primary care team members will help to assist and sustain this shift in perspective and care.

A parallel shift in perspective is needed in the community. Community education and advocacy are needed to increase awareness about common signs and symptoms of mental health disorders, the availability of successful treatments, and the importance of practitioners inquiring about patient stress, health behaviors, and reactions to illnesses.

This inter-country consultation team has experienced significant reciprocity. The consultation has been a two-way process. The Vietnamese co-authors, colleagues, and learners inform the US consultants about the Vietnamese health system, culture, and psychosocial dimensions of illness, care, and health-seeking behaviors. The US consultants inform the Vietnamese about behavioral medicine and mental healthcare through what we have learned from the successes and struggles in our systems. These discussions help to prioritize content, provide vision, and determine how best to fit behavioral medicine into their cultural and community milieu. The aim is to serve as a resource for information that will complement traditional and current beliefs and practices.

This project is national in scope, operating in several diverse communities in Vietnam. Each regional training program and its faculty vary in their views about best teaching practices, readiness to address social issues such as alcohol abuse or family violence, and access to behavioral medicine resources for teaching and mental healthcare. The cultures of the patient populations differ according to geographical location, degree of urbanization, and economic resources. For example, the Thai Nguyen program has physicians practicing in mountain communities with many ethnic minorities and a high level of poverty. The communities on the coast have higher concentrations of intravenous drug users and commercial sex workers. Communities in the Mekong Delta region close to Cambodia tend to have a high rate of human sex trafficking.

These intercultural conversations have taken place in the USA and in Vietnam. Funding has supported 30 Vietnamese faculty physicians to travel to the USA, giving them exposure to two or more US training sites to see how our culture integrates behavioral medicine into family medicine education and treatment. Annual visits of US faculty to Vietnam have included psychiatrists, social workers, and sociologists.

Faculty teams conduct 2-week Behavioral Medicine Certificate courses to train faculty from departments of family medicine, public health, nursing, social work, and pharmacy. The course is very practical and experiential, using lectures, demonstrations, role play, small group work, case discussions, individual exercises, and family sculpting. Topics have been organized around the major content areas of this book. The application and appropriate fine-tuning of behavioral medicine principles and practices for the Vietnamese context depends on how well practitioners and these newly trained teachers incorporate these principles and skills into their care.[20]

PROJECTS IN OTHER RESOURCE-CONSTRAINED COUNTRIES

Many others are working to incorporate mental health and behavioral health principles into primary care training and practice in resource-constrained countries. Consulting US physicians report varying degrees of success in influencing training in the doctor–patient relationship and in diagnosing serious mental health problems. The financial domain determines, in large part, the extent to which mental health and behavioral health services can be integrated into primary healthcare (the operational domain). Countries that are experiencing environmental catastrophes, war, or other violence also confront chaotic healthcare systems and an increase in the number of people experiencing trauma reactions, calling for even more mental health services. In the clinical domain, providing patient care with learners present is often where behavioral medicine skills are modeled, triggering discussions about how medical practitioners express culturally appropriate caring, empathy, and relationship-centered care.

In the cultural domain, the standard of patient care often parallels the teaching and culture, and this is particularly evident in settings that support a paternalistic, autocratic mode of decision making. Women from around the world have experienced neglect and both verbal and physical abuse in healthcare settings.[21] They have cited fears of being hit, shouted at, denigrated, or dismissed as reasons for not seeking care during childbirth.[22]

In resource-constrained countries, the teaching of communication and other behavioral medicine skills is often demonstrated by using a mentoring teaching model by family physicians who stay in-country for concentrated periods of time (clinical/teaching domain). Modeling, case-based discussions, and care plans become opportunities for conducting healthy dialogues about outcomes for success related to doctor–patient interactions. Unique teaching challenges exist for out-of-country consultants in countries where the beliefs and values are directly opposed to their own. This is where cultural humility and curiosity, not pedantic opposition, are required.

Table 10.2 depicts mental health/primary healthcare integration projects in countries of varying economic levels. Projects in low-income countries (Belize and South Africa) have specially trained nurses who provide training, consultation, and care to the primary healthcare practitioners. Projects in moderate-income countries (Uganda, Iran, Brazil, and Chile) incorporate case finding by community health workers, collaboration with community mental health and substance abuse centers, and consultation and training by psychiatrists and professional counselors. Projects in high-income countries (Saudi Arabia and the UK) incorporate group and individual counseling by mental health specialists and formal relationships with community organizations on employment, housing, and legal issues.

TABLE 10.2 Best practice sites and statistics for integrating mental healthcare into primary care

Country	World Bank income group	Gross national income*	% of GDP spent on health	Project sites and descriptions of care for people with mental illnesses
Uganda	Low	1500	7.6	*Sanbabule District:* Primary care doctors diagnose and treat. Specialist outreach teams consult, train, and supervise. Village health teams identify, refer, and provide follow-up.
Vietnam	Low	2490	4	*Khanh Hoa Province:* Psychiatrists in district hospitals are referral sources to diagnose and treat people from surrounding communities.
India	Low	3460	5	*Thiravananthapuram District, Kerala State:* Medical officers diagnose and treat at community level. District mental health team provides outreach, manages complex cases, provides in-service training, and supervises medical officers.
Iran	Low–middle	8050	6.6	*Nationwide:* General doctors assess and treat. Complex cases are referred to district or provincial health centers. Treatment is mostly medications, disease management, and secondary prevention. Community health workers (*behvarzes*) case find and refer.
Belize	Upper–middle	6740	5.1	*Nationwide:* Psychiatric nurse practitioners in district health centers train primary care doctors and staff, consult, and see patients in their homes. Uses a two-tiered approach, utilizing nurses until the mental health skills of primary healthcare team are suitable.

(*continued*)

Country	World Bank income group	Gross national income*	% of GDP spent on health	Project sites and descriptions of care for people with mental illnesses
Brazil	Upper–middle	8230	8.8	*City of Sobrol:* Primary care doctors assess and treat. Specialist mobile mental health teams routinely visit to consult, train, and discuss cases. Mental health workers identify patients. Group treatment and support available.
Chile	Upper–middle	11,470	6.1	*Macul District of Santiago:* Primary care doctors assess and treat. Psychologists provide individual, family, and group treatment. Staff from mental health community centers consult, supervise, and treat. Volunteer workers identify and refer.
South Africa	Upper–middle	12,120	8.6	*Ehlanzeni District, Mpumalanga Province:* Two options exist: (1) psychiatric nurses see all mental health patients; (2) primary care workers diagnose and treat mental health disorders.
South Africa	Upper–middle	12,120	8.6	*Moorreesburg District, Western Cape Province:* Primary care nurses assess and treat. Psychiatric nurses visit monthly to manage complex cases and supervise. Regional psychiatrists visit every 3 months. Psychologists see patients for 8 hours a week.
Argentina	High	13,920	9.6	*Province of Neuquen:* Primary care doctors diagnose and treat. Psychiatrists consult. Community rehabilitation centers treat patients.
Saudi Arabia	High	14,740	3.9	*Eastern Province, Ash-Sharqiyah:* Primary care doctors diagnose and treat. Primary care doctors with specialized training treat complex cases. Community mental health clinics provide rehabilitation, medication, and psychotherapy. Secondary and tertiary treatment centers are available.
Australia	High	30,610	9.6	*Inner-city Sydney:* Care for the mental health needs of older people: primary care doctors diagnose and treat. Psychogeriatric nurses, psychologists, and psychiatrists consult.

Country	World Bank income group	Gross national income*	% of GDP spent on health	Project sites and descriptions of care for people with mental illnesses
UK	High	33,650	8.2	*London:* Disadvantaged communities project: primary care doctors diagnose, treat, and refer to formal and volunteer community services to help with employment, housing, and legal issues.

* Gross national income equated in US$.

Adapted from World Health Organization. *WHO/Wonca Joint Report: integrating mental health into primary care – a global perspective*; www.who.int/mental_health/policy/Mental%20health%20+%20 primary%20care-%20final%20low-res%20140908.pdf (accessed 3 April 2009).

RECOMMENDED STRATEGIES

Table 10.3 shows strategies for incorporating behavioral health interventions in rural communities, based on the work of Rahman and colleagues with Pakistani mothers and children (*see* Chapter 6). These strategies are focused on the clinical domain, and clearly take into consideration the cultural domain and aspects of care described in Chapter 6.

TABLE 10.3 Strategies to consider when designing rural behavioral health interventions for perinatal depression

Intervention level	Healthcare practitioner strategy
Patient/family level	<ul><li>Focus on infant and maternal health, not maternal depression</li><li>Make interventions active and empowering</li><li>Make intervention participatory for mothers</li><li>Consider existing family roles and responsibilities</li></ul>
Health worker level	<ul><li>Integrate worker into existing system where possible</li><li>Develop simple step-by-step interventions that are easily delivered</li><li>Be aware of potential stigmatization of mothers in the program</li></ul>
Health system level	<ul><li>Make it evidence based</li><li>Avoid a strict adherence to the "medical model"</li><li>Provide home- or community-based services</li><li>Adapt materials to local culture(s)</li><li>Be aware of limitations of existing health systems</li></ul>

Adapted from Rahman A. Challenges and opportunities in developing a psychological intervention for perinatal depression in rural Pakistan – a multi-method study. *Arch Womens Ment Health.* 2007; **10:** 213.

The WHO and Wonca have developed key strategies to guide the integration of mental healthcare into primary care, regardless of a country's economic status, culture, or political system, or the presence of national trauma.[23] These strategies can easily incorporate behavioral healthcare as well. They are compatible with the four-world view of systems development, specified in parentheses after each principle described below.

1 **Policies and plans must incorporate primary care for mental health on a national scale** and at every level of the healthcare system (*policy and operational domains*). The work in Vietnam related to family medicine and social work is closely aligned with the appropriate ministries of health, education, and social affairs, in order to facilitate the approval of new schools of study and new curricula, the creation of new jobs, and the setting of new pay structures.

2 **Advocacy is required** to shift attitudes and behaviors. This includes advocacy directed toward legislators, public officials, healthcare practitioners, and the general public about the benefits of treatment and the economic, social, and healthcare costs of no treatment of mental and behavioral health conditions (*all four domains*). We have introduced behavioral medicine principles into our consultation early and often. At the same time, we have tried to balance this advocacy with a stance of cultural humility, openly acknowledging that out-of-country advisors do not know what is "best" for a country's medical system. Our Vietnamese co-authors, Pham Huy Dung, MD, PhD, and Nguyen Thi Kim Chuc, PhD, have been tireless advocates at a national level for incorporating mental and behavioral healthcare into medical training and primary healthcare. Many of our Vietnamese chapter co-authors have done the same in their local and regional communities.

3 **Adequate training is required** for primary care workers in the epidemiology, evidence-based guidelines, and skills necessary to treat mental and behavioral health conditions (*clinical domain*). In Vietnam, we have worked at incorporating this training into all levels of administration and care, including students, practitioners, administrators, and managers.

4 **Primary care tasks must be limited and feasible** (*clinical domain*), as they are highly dependent on financial resources (*see* Table 10.2) (*financial domain*).

5 **Specialist mental health professionals and facilities must be available**, because the provision of mental healthcare in primary care cannot be sustained without supervision and support (*clinical and operational domains*). In most of Vietnam, psychiatrists are available at the district or provincial levels of care. Community mental health and substance abuse services are typically not accessible in the majority of communities, and the same is true for professional mental health counselors.

6 **Patients must have access to essential psychotropic medication** in primary care. Primary care integration projects have struggled wherever access to psychotropic medication has been limited or such medication has been inconsistently available (*operational domain*).

7 **Integration is a process, not an event.** This process will not happen overnight, but will take time (*all four domains*). As we have seen in Belize, a phased-in approach to integration can be practical and realistic, particularly when psychiatrists and specialty mental health therapists are not available. In Vietnam,

we have seen projects at different sites develop at different paces and in different ways, depending on the extent to which professional resources are available.

8 **A mental health service coordinator is crucial** at the national and local levels (*operational domain*). We have sought out informal and formal leaders to inspire and to be inspired to take action. The success of specific sites has been dependent on the level of interest and advocacy taken by particular faculty members. At this point in time, there is no formal coordinator identified by the government to direct the integration of mental health and behavioral healthcare into primary care.

9 **Collaboration with other government non-health sectors, non-government organizations (NGOs), community health workers, and volunteers is an absolute necessity** (*financial, operational, and cultural domains*). In Vietnam, our training and strategizing has been informed and has benefited tremendously by collaborating with others from international government agencies, NGOs, and community organizations. We have sought out and listened to the views of in-country and out-of-country advisors. The perspectives of in-country teachers, administrators, and practitioners have often differed from those of out-of-country medical practitioners, community members, or international medical school graduates training in the USA.

10 **Financial and human resources are needed** (*financial domain*). The Vietnam project continues to pursue funding from government and non-government organizations to improve the overall health of its population through the integration of mental health and behavioral health services into its primary healthcare system.

CONCLUSION

Our Vietnam project has influenced the country's advancement of behavioral health and mental health integration into primary care training and practice. It has helped to transform the Vietnamese primary healthcare system, by paying attention to the four domains of clinical care/teaching, operations, finance/policy, and culture. Factors contributing to the project's success include the hard work of our in-country colleagues, the vision of the US–Vietnamese team, funding that has supported a continuous relationship between advisory team members, a progressive Ministry of Health, and Vietnam's rapidly expanding economy.

Conducting behavioral medicine consultations in countries other than one's own can be challenging. By using the four-domain model, the similarities and differences between a Western model and another country's model of teaching and care can be more clearly understood. Behavioral medicine is a powerful and necessary component for any international healthcare consultation, providing transformational tools that can improve the overall functioning and health of patients, communities, and healthcare systems. Our hope is that these experiences will contribute to the success of others in advancing behavioral medicine and mental health services in developing areas of the world.

KEY RESOURCE

● World Health Organization. *WHO/Wonca Joint Report: integrating mental health into primary care – a global perspective*; www.who.int/mental_health/policy/Mental%20health%20+%20primary%20care-%20final%20low-res%20140908.pdf (accessed 3 April 2009).

REFERENCES

1 Patel V, Araya R, Chatterjee S, *et al.* Treatment and prevention of mental disorders in low-income and middle-income countries. *Lancet.* 2007; **370**: 991–1005.

2 Desjarlais R, Eisenberg L, Good B, *et al. World Mental Health: problems and priorities in low-income countries.* Oxford: Oxford University Press, Inc; 1995.

3 Kramer M. The rising pandemic of mental disorders and associated chronic diseases and disabilities. *Acta Psychiatr Scand.* 2007; **62**: 382–97.

4 Cross-National Collaborative Group. The changing rate of major depression. *JAMA.* 1992; **268**: 3098–105.

5 World Health Organization. *Best Practices – Mental Health Services: primary care*; www.who.int/mental_health/policy/country/BestPractices8_SEARO.pdf (accessed 3 April 2008).

6 Nishtar S, Minhas FA, Ahmed A, *et al.* Prevention and control of mental illness and mental health: National Action Plan for NCD Prevention, Control and Health Promotion in Pakistan. *J Pak Med Assoc.* 2004; **54(Suppl. 3)**: S69–77.

7 Montegut AJ, Cartwright C, Schirmer JM, *et al.* An international consultation: the development of family medicine education in Vietnam. *Fam Med.* 2004; **35**: 352–6.

8 Schirmer JM, Cartwright C, Montegut AJ, *et al.* A collaborative needs assessment and work plan in behavioral medicine curriculum development in Vietnam. *Fam Syst Health.* 2005; **22**: 410–18.

9 Schirmer J, Ninh LH. The Vietnam family medicine development project: a cross-cultural collaboration. *Fam Syst Health.* 2002; **20**: 303–10.

10 World Bank. *Country Classification of Economy*; http://web.worldbank.org/WBSITE/EXTERNAL/DATASTATISTICS/0,contentMDK:20420458~menuPK:64133156~pagePK:64133150~piPK:64133175~theSitePK:239419,00.html (accessed 4 April 2008).

11 Collins P. Half-way from rags to riches (special report on Vietnam). *Economist.* 2008; **387**: 3–5.

12 Healy J, Scalzo F, Tam MN. *Poverty and Health: the poor of Phong Thu Commune, Phong Dien District, Thua Thien Hué Province, Vietnam.* Hué, Vietnam: Hué Medical School; 2006.

13 Pham L. Personal communication. 2007.

14 Family Health International. *Family Health International Programs: FHI takes a three-prong approach*; www.fhi.org/en/HIVAIDS/country/VietNam/vietnamprograms.htm (accessed 4 April 2008).

15 Kleinman A. *Patients and Healers in the Context of Culture: an exploration of the borderland between anthropology, medicine, and psychiatry.* Berkeley, CA: University of California Press; 1980.

16 Schwartz PY. Why is neurasthenia important in Asian cultures? *West J Med.* 2002; **176**: 257–8.

17 Thach TD, Ha TT, Tuan T, *et al. Assessing and Modeling Community Mental Health and Rehabilitation in Da Nang and Khanh Hoa Provinces: Final Report.* Hanoi, Vietnam: Vietnam Veterans of America Foundation Mental Health Program; 2007.

18 Peek CJ, Heinrich R. Building a collaborative healthcare organization: from idea to invention to innovation. *Fam Syst Health*. 1995; **13**: 327–42.
19 Feldman MD, Christensen JF. *Behavioral Medicine in Primary Care: a practical guide*. Stanford, CT: Appleton & Lange; 1997.
20 Candib LM, Stovall JG. Response to Schirmer and Le (Medical Family Therapy Casebook). *Fam Syst Health*. 2002; **20**: 419–28.
21 d'Oliveira AF, Diniz SG, Schraiber LB. Violence against women in health-care institutions: an emerging problem. *Lancet*. 2002; **359**: 1681–5.
22 Rothenberg D. Personal communication. 2007.
23 World Health Organization. *WHO/Wonca Joint Report: integrating mental health into primary care – a global perspective*; www.who.int/mental_health/policy/Mental%20health%20+%20primary%20care-%20final%20low-res%20140908.pdf (accessed 3 April 2009).

Glossary of terms

Acceptance	holding positive attitudes towards, acknowledging, and accepting of human differences
Action stage	the stage at which a patient has the vision, motivation, skills, and plan to change their behavior to improve their health
Actualization	holding the belief that people, groups, and society have potential and can evolve or grow positively
Acute	(of a medical disease) having severe symptoms and a short course
Adherence	remaining steadily on a treatment regimen
Affect	disposition, feeling, and tendency
Agonist	something that produces an action; a drug that binds to a cell and produces a response in the cell; often mimics nature
Ailment	sickness, lack of health
Algorithm	a step-by-step way of solving a problem
Align	to bring into line
Alliance	a positive relationship or close connection between people, families, or groups, often in order to further the mutual interests of all involved
Ancillary	something subordinate or subservient to something else
Antagonist	acting against and blocking an action
Anxiety	a condition characterized by feeling tense, worried, keyed up, or on edge
Autonomy	independence; being guided by one's own, socially accepted, internal standards and values
Ayurvedic	an approach to healthcare based on Hindu principles of maintaining balance between the five elements of earth, air, fire, water, and ether. It involves diet, massage, yoga, and herbs
Balint group	a group of health or social service practitioners who present cases in order to increase their understanding of what they bring to the encounter that is either helpful or harmful to the patient

Behavioralist	a professional caregiver who values and has skills to address the biological, psychological, social, and spiritual factors that affect a person's health
Bias	a preference or inclination towards an object or view
Biopsychosocial model	a model that considers the possible biological, emotional, familial, social, and spiritual contributions and solutions to patients' symptoms and illnesses
Boundary	that which defines the different functional subgroups in the family; a border or limit
Burnout	a syndrome characterized by emotional exhaustion, cynicism, and low personal achievement
Chronic	(of a medical disease) of long duration
Coalition	a temporary union; a relationship between at least three people in which two act together secretly against a third person
Coercion	bringing about an event or situation by threats, intimidation, or force
Cognitive–behavioral therapy	a form of counseling that helps to change unhealthy patterns of thinking or behaving into healthy patterns
Coherence	(as in social coherence) a state in which one is interested in society and social life and finds them meaningful and somewhat intelligible
Communal	pertaining to a commune; belonging to or shared by a particular community
Compassion fatigue	a deep physical, emotional, and spiritual exhaustion accompanied by acute emotional pain
Consultation	the act of consulting or conferring; deliberation of two or more physicians about diagnosis or treatment in a particular case with a view to reaching a decision
Contemplative stage	the stage at which patients consider making the changes necessary to improve their health
Culturally derived syndrome	physical symptoms with a prescribed psychiatric component that presents in an idiosyncratic way particular to a culture or geographic region
Curious	eager for knowledge, anxious to learn, habitually inquisitive
Curriculum	a specified fixed course of study
Denigrate	to speak ill of; to defame
Depersonalization	a feeling of detachment from one's work, one's family, and one's own emotional experience
Depression	a condition characterized by feeling hopeless and helpless, and lacking interest in things, which affects a person's functioning for 2 months or more
Differentiate	to discriminate or show the differences in or between
Disband	to cease to function as an organization or group

Discrepancy	the difference between one's beliefs that contribute to unhealthy choices and the evidence that challenges such beliefs
Disease	the malfunctioning of biological or disease processes
Disengagement	release from one's relationships or obligations; a situation in which family members are emotionally distant and unresponsive to one another
Dispensary	a place where drugs or medicines are dispensed
Empathy	willingness to understand another's situation, feelings, or motives
Enmeshment	the entanglement of family members with one another, as in a mesh
Environmental mastery	exercising the ability to select, manage, and mold one's personal environment to meet one's needs
Epidemiology	the study of the causes, distribution, and control of various diseases in populations
Etiology	the study of the causes or origins of disease
Explicit	clearly defined and observable
External locus of control	the perception that one's fate is determined outside of oneself; the belief that one has little control over one's life
Extrovert	a person who is gregarious and who feels renewed by spending time with many people
Flourishing	having high levels of emotional well-being, psychological functioning, and social functioning
Fortune teller	a person who claims to be able to predict events in the future of another person
Hallucination	the phenomenon whereby a person sees or hears things that others cannot see or hear
Hierarchy	the way in which power or authority is distributed within the family; any of a series of clearly organized rankings or grades
Humility	the state of being humble; freedom from pride and arrogance
Illness	the experience and meaning of perceived disease
Implicit	implied or inferred without being expressly stated
Impulse control disorders	inability to resist an impulsive act or behavior that may be harmful to one's self or others
Index	that which points out, shows, indicates, manifests, or discloses
Indigenous	occurring naturally within an area or culture
Inefficacy	feelings of lack of personal achievement, loss of control over one's life, and failure
Insomnia	difficulty with sleeping
Integration	the act of bringing components together in order to unify them; (social integration) a sense of belonging

	to, and of deriving comfort and support from, a community
Interdisciplinary	including two or more professional disciplines in the provision of care
Internal locus of control	the perception that one's fate is determined by one's actions; the belief that one is in control of one's life and destiny
Interpersonal therapy	a form of counseling that helps to identify unhealthy patterns of relating to one's family, friends, and colleagues
Introvert	a person who is shy and who feels renewed by spending time alone or with very few people
Maintenance stage	the stage at which patients are able to sustain healthy behaviors that they have developed in order to improve their health
Malpractice	improper or unethical behavior by professional caregivers
Manifestation	the indication that something is real, evident, or present
Metaphor	a symbol, whereby one thing denotes another
Milieu	one's surroundings or environment
Mnemonic	a device, such as a rhyme or word, that is used as an aid to memory
Motivational interviewing	a form of counseling in which the practitioner relates to the patient in a way that matches the patient's readiness to change, in order to inspire them to make the changes necessary to improve their health
Neurasthenia	a condition that I characterized by chronic fatigue, memory problems, aches and pains
Neuropsychiatry	the study of disorders that pertain to the relationship between the nervous system and mental and emotional functions
Nomenclature	technical terms that are used in any particular branch of science or art
On-site	taking place or located at the indicated site
Overriding	more important than other factors
Panic	a condition of severe anxiety in which the affected person feels that they are going to die. It is usually characterized by difficulty in breathing, and can lead to avoidance of situations that may trigger the condition
Pedantic	narrowly and boastfully learned; making a vain display of learning
Perceived criticism	the perception by family members that their opinions or contributions are not valued; the perception that others find one at fault and are judgmental about this

Personal growth	the process whereby one seeks challenges, gains insight into one's own potential, and feels a sense of ongoing development
Pervade	to permeate; to be diffused throughout
Placebo	a substance containing no medication that is given in order to appease a person or condition (instead of giving them a real drug)
Pluralistic	believing that no single view of reality accounts for all phenomena (as in the cause and treatment of disease)
Postpartum depression	a condition characterized by feelings of intense sadness that occurs within 3 months of having a baby
Post-traumatic stress disorder (PTSD)	a condition characterized by panic, anxiety, and the re-experiencing of traumatic feelings and sensations after a life-threatening event or series of events
Precontemplative stage	the stage at which a patient is unaware of or denies the severity of the contribution of their behaviors to their health issues
Preparation stage	the stage at which patients have the vision to change, but do not yet have the skills necessary to make the changes that are needed to improve their health
Prevention	anticipation and action to impede or stop something from happening
Progressive	moving forward in continuous steady increments
Prophylaxis	measures taken to prevent ill health or to preserve health
Prosthesis	an artificial device that is used to replace a missing body part, such as a limb or a tooth
Psychiatry	the branch of medicine that deals with the study, treatment, and prevention of mental illness
Psychosomatic	referring to a condition in which physical symptoms are caused by emotional and psychological stressors
Psychotropic	exerting an effect on the mind (e.g. psychotropic drugs)
Relapse	return to a problem behavior, after sustained resolution of that behavior
Relational context of symptoms	a symptom seen as a part of a larger family and psychosocial context that can influence and be influenced by that symptom
Resilience	the ability to recover from or adjust to misfortune or change
Resistance	the ability to oppose or counteract; the ability to fight a disease
Role	the characteristics or behavior expected of an individual (e.g. the conscious or unconscious assignment of complementary roles to members of a family)

Self-acceptance	the demonstration of positive attitudes towards oneself, acknowledging and liking most aspects of self and personality
Self-efficacy	the belief that one is able to make the changes necessary to improve one's health
Social contribution	daily activities that are useful to and valued by others
Somatic	referring to the body as a whole; corporeal; characteristic of the body
Somatoform	referring to general physical symptoms, such as pain, nausea, or dizziness, which have no organic cause, usually accompanied by intense worry and concern about the symptoms
Stability	an interpersonal process by which family members strive to maintain emotional balance in the system
Stance	mental attitude, position
Stigmatize	to regard as disgraceful or not important
Stressor	a condition, situation, or other stimulus that causes extreme difficulty, pressure, or pain
Syndrome	a cluster of symptoms
Transition	an interpersonal process by which the family adapts to developmental growth of its members, and to varying expectations and roles in the community
Trauma	a wound or injury, especially damage caused by external force
Worldview	the general view that family members have of themselves as competent or ineffective, cohesive or fragmented

Index

psychosomatic complaints 71, 147
psychotropic medication 9, 132, 138, 147
public health 4, 42
public health model 2–3

qi (vital energy) 31
quality of life 113, 123

Rahe, RH 10
Rahman, A 137
recognition 120–1
reframing thoughts 34, 35, 74, 75
refugees 69, 70, 89
rehabilitation programs 95
reimbursement parity 69
relapse 47, 48, 50–1, 88, 95, 118, 147
relational context of illness 54, 55, 56, 147
relationship building 25
relationship-centered care 4, 7, 134
relative poverty 128
relaxation response 32
relaxation techniques 91, 94, 107
resilience 120, 123, 147
resistance 47, 49, 147
risk reduction counseling 44–5
role (definition) 147
role selection 56, 57
Rollnick, Stephen 51
rural behavioral health interventions 137

sanitation 5, 78
Saudi Arabia 135, 136
schizophrenia 8, 95
Scrimshaw, SC 72
secondary care 86
secondary trauma 102
sedatives 90
selective serotonin reuptake inhibitors (SSRIs) 90, 94
self-acceptance 113, 148
self-efficacy 4–5, 43, 46, 47, 148
self-management plans 106–7
Selye, Hans 32
sexual abuse 102
sexual behavior 8, 41, 46, 47
sex workers 44, 46, 47, 133
shamans 2, 36, 74
Shanghai, China 127
shenjing shuairou (neurasthenia) 31
shock 72
sleep hygiene 92, 93, 100
sleeping sickness 86
sleep problems
    mental health in primary care 86, 88, 89, 91–3, 94

practitioner well-being 114, 119, 121, 123
smoking
    behavioral change 3, 8, 12, 41, 44–5, 48–51
    mental health in primary care 85, 93
    practitioner well-being 115, 118
snake healers 36
social acceptance 113
social actualization 113
social coherence 113
social contribution 113, 148
social functioning 112, 113
social influences 68–81
    alternative ways of conceptualizing health and care 72–5
    biopsychosocial model 21
    case scenarios 68, 71, 72, 74, 75, 76
    community-oriented primary care 77–8
    culturally sensitive healthcare 78–9
    disease versus illness 71–2
    ethnocentrism 75–7
    finding common ground with patients 38
    importance of culture 69–70
    insider versus outsider perspectives 70–1
    key resources 81
    overview 69, 80
    preparing to work in healthcare settings in a different culture 79–80
    principles and practices of behavioral medicine 11–12
social integration 113
social phobia 90
social sphere 23
social work 36, 37, 132, 138
Society of Behavioral Medicine 15
Society of Teachers of Family Medicine (STFM) 4, 81
somatic (definition) 148
somatization disorder 31
somatoform disorders 91, 148
South Africa 134, 136
South America 127
spirituality 36, 71
stability 148
stages of change 8, 46–9, 143, 144, 146, 147
stance (definition) 148
stigma 85, 116, 127, 129
stigmatize (definition) 148
stress 29–40
    brief supportive counseling 104
    case scenarios 29
    cognitive therapy 33–5